Ready...Set...Advocate!

Your Step-by-Step Guide to Patient Empowerment

Randy Sperling

Lorrie Klemons, RN, MSN

To order more books, visit **ReadySetAdvocate.com.**

The information contained in this book is not meant to diagnose or treat any health-related issues or to replace the advice of a doctor. Speak to your personal health care provider about any symptoms you are experiencing. Patient Action disclaims any liability for the decisions you make based on this information.

First published by Dog Ear Publishing
4011 Vincennes Rd
Indianapolis, IN 46268
www.dogearpublishing.net

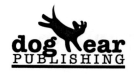

ISBN: 978-1-4575-4612-9

This book is printed on acid-free paper.

Printed in the United States of America

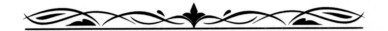

In Memory of Philip Joshua Sperling,
whose kind heart and sweet soul
inspired the creation of Patient Action

~February 23, 1970–January 2, 2011~

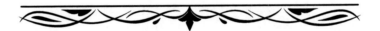

Table of Contents

ABOUT THE BOOK

Patient Advocacy is the process of acting to ensure that a patient is served adequately by the health care system.

A Patient Advocate is the person who ensures that the patient is served adequately by the health care system by promoting the cause, safeguarding the rights, and supporting the interests of that patient.

You or someone you care about has probably been a patient in a health care setting at some time. Often, that setting can be complex and scary. Making sure you have a voice and are being served adequately by the health care system is essential to achieving the best health care outcomes possible. Regardless of your age or condition, when you become a patient, you need a patient advocate to make sure your voice will be heard ... especially if you are unable to speak for yourself because you are scared, confused, anxious, in pain, unconscious, under the influence of certain drugs or other substances, under anesthesia, physically or mentally unable to speak, or unable to speak the local language.

As a nurse and nurse educator, coauthor Lorrie Klemons spent the first thirty-nine years of her career advocating for her patients and teaching others to do the same. Co-author Randy Sperling spent more than twenty-five years advocating for her sick son, Philip. When Lorrie and Randy met in 2008, they realized that they not only shared a heart but also shared a passion for patient advocacy. As a result of their collective passion and the constant encouragement from Philip, they created this step-by-step guide to patient advocacy and empowerment. This book will guide you as you navigate through any health care setting.

Finding your voice and using it to partner with the health care team so you can advocate for yourself or someone you care about in the health care setting can be stressful if you don't have much medical knowledge to guide you. With the purchase of this book, you have taken a major step in finding your voice and becoming an empowered patient advocate. **CONGRATULATIONS!**

You can also join Lorrie and Randy at __PatientAction.com__, their website dedicated to making sure that every patient's voice is heard in the health care setting through patient empowerment and advocacy. Philip's untimely death in January 2011 became the inspiration to making that creation what it is today—the premier site for patient advocacy. **YOU HAVE A VOICE ... Use it!**

ABOUT PATIENT ACTION

Patient Action was created by co-authors Lorrie Klemons and Randy Sperling as a result of their collective passion for and exploration into patient advocacy and empowerment. The mission of Patient Action is to help you find your voice as you partner with the health care team in a *positive* way to get the best health care outcomes possible for yourself or any loved one you may be advocating for.

Lorrie and Randy invite you to visit the **free** resources on **www.PatientAction.com**, designed to educate and empower you in a variety of health care settings.

Advocacy articles, many of which correlate with the worksheets contained in this book, provide you with the information you need to advocate for yourself or someone you care about.

The Resources section offers wonderful useful tips, current health news, links to reliable medical information websites, and an interactive community blog, which you are invited to participate in.

The Inspirational section offers prayers, inspirational sayings, and an interactive place for you to share your own advocacy stories, prayers, and inspirational sayings in the hopes of inspiring other members of the Patient Action community.

A key benefit of being part of the Patient Action community is that you also have access to patient advocates through live one-on-one telephone and online advocacy coaching at a fee-for-service rate. These coaches will personally guide you through your journey to help you find your voice. Visit **PatientAction.com** for information on how to access these coaching services, or email **info@patientaction.com**. Lorrie and Randy are also available to speak at your next group meeting.

YOU HAVE A VOICE…USE IT!

The Authors' Stories

Lorrie Klemons

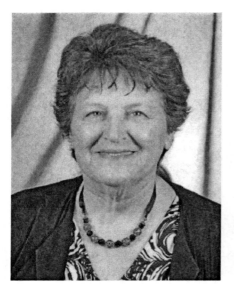

I was exposed to nursing at the age of four when my thirty-two-year-old mother became a victim of the polio epidemic in the early 1950s. Although too young to remember many details, I do remember the ladies in white who made my mother feel so good and gave her reason to smile. At the age of fifteen, I spent the summer as a candy striper volunteer at our local hospital, and that experience solidified my choice to become a nurse. I knew it was my destiny.

During my four years at the Hunter College-Bellevue School of Nursing, many of the patients I cared for were indigent. Few spoke English. Few had family or friends who cared. I quickly realized that these patients did not have a voice and had no one to speak for them. They frequently did not get the care they needed.. or deserved.

What could I do to make it better? How could I make a difference? I decided to go to graduate school and become a nurse educator. If I couldn't change the system, I could at least change the product. I could educate nurses who cared, who advocated for their patients, and who practiced their chosen occupation with integrity, caring, and professionalism.

Earning a master's degree in nursing has opened many doors for me. I have had a wonderful career in the nursing and education arena. Over the span of my nursing and teaching career, I have touched many lives, and I know that I have made a difference ... as a nurse, as an educator, and as a patient advocate.

I spent the first thirty-nine years of my career obsessed with making sure that patients received the great nursing care that they deserved. Now I am on a new journey—the journey to help patients find their voices, the journey to help patients achieve the best health care outcomes possible by partnering with their health care team in a positive way. Over the course of my career, I have been witness to the individual's loss of identity, dignity, and control upon entrance to the health care setting, but that doesn't need to be a patient's reality anymore, as the mission of this book revolutionizes the patient experience. No longer must patients be uninformed non-participants in their own care. No longer must they agree to things they don't understand. No longer must they allow strangers to make the decisions that may alter their lives forever. The goal of PatientAction.com is to help patients find their voice ... and use it! This goal can be achieved through the guidance from our new step-by-step guide to patient empowerment.

Addendum: In March, 2016, all of my professional experience and best mothering strategies were called into action when my 32 year-old son was diagnosed with two concurrent life threatening conditions at the same time. I spent 47 days at my son's hospital bedside and was with him 24/7 for seven terrorizing months. While I'm happy to report my son's story has a very happy ending, this experience has impassioned me even more in the work I do, assuring that every patient's voice is heard.

Randy Sperling

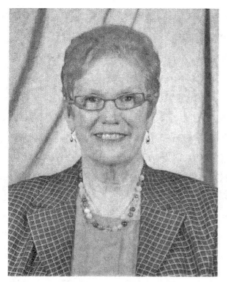

My family was in the midst of a busy 1985 summer with baseball, sleepovers, camping, and friends in and out of the house. My husband and I felt blessed as our three sons were growing into model teens. Life was busy, but uncomplicated. Then our eldest son, Philip, required an appointment with an endocrinologist one July morning. I was horrified when the doctor diagnosed a possible brain tumor. I called my husband and told him to meet us at the hospital. I called my business partner and told him I would be unavailable. I called a friend and asked her to pray. That day was full of doctors, tests, anxiety, and confusion. I quickly found myself in an alien world, and all I could do was watch and cooperate. I didn't know my life would change forever that day as I assumed the role of patient advocate.

Even having worked in several healthcare settings, I was totally unprepared for the task of becoming Philip's advocate. Through a process of trial and error, desperation and creativity, I learned how to navigate and manage the health care system so my son received the best care possible throughout his twenty-five-year illness. I learned how to research medical diagnoses and procedures. I learned how to research relevant clinical trials. I learned how to research prescribed drugs to understand the benefits, risks, complications, and drug interactions. I learned how a hospital operates and how to make it work to my advantage. I learned about alternative treatments such as acupuncture, massage, and herbs, etc. I learned the questions to ask at a doctor's appointment, before a test or procedure. I learned how to navigate through insurance companies to get approval for the services my son needed. I asked questions and confirmed information so I always had a clear understanding of what was happening and why. I learned to remain calm and polite so I could become a positive influence in working with Philip's health care team.

Philip's journey was a difficult one, but having me as his patient advocate gave him tremendous peace of mind. He knew that my advocacy gave him a huge advantage over other patients. Philip initiated our first end-of-life conversation before he turned sixteen. He wanted us to be open and honest with him. He didn't want to live in a vegetative state. After dozens of hospitalizations, radiation therapy, three strokes, and, eventually, liver failure caused by the medication that kept him alive, he lost his twenty-five-year battle in 2011. Our family misses him terribly every day; however, we are all at peace knowing that as his patient advocate, I was able to get him the best care possible.

Philip always encouraged me to help others with their advocacy issues. This book is the result of his encouragement and belief that every person benefits from patient advocacy.

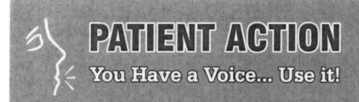

ACUTE/EMERGENCY CARE

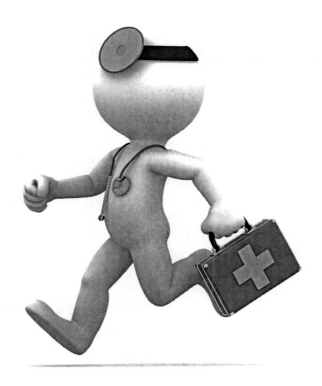

IN CASE OF MEDICAL EMERGENCY

When do I need to go to the emergency room (ER)? How do I get there? What happens once I am there?

A medical emergency is when:

❑ The absence of medical care can result in serious impairment to bodily function.

❑ The absence of medical care can result in serious dysfunction of any bodily organ or part.

❑ The absence of medical care can result in serious jeopardy to the health of the individual or unborn child.

**If you do have a medical emergency: Call 911.
Do not drive yourself or be driven to the ER in a car, bus, or taxi.**

Call 911 for the following symptoms:

❑ Chest pain, suspected heart attack

❑ Difficulty breathing

❑ Severe and persistent abdominal pain

❑ Uncontrolled or excessive bleeding

❑ Head injury

❑ Loss of consciousness

❑ Poisoning (after you've called the Poison Control hotline at 1-800-222-1222)

❑ Severe burn

❑ High fever over 103 degrees, especially in children

❑ Seizures

❑ Diabetic complications such an insulin shock or ketoacidosis

❑ Gunshot or stab wounds

What to bring with you to the ER:

❑ Patient Advocate ... or have one meet you at the ER. Allow your advocate to speak for you when necessary.

❑ Completed health history (include allergies, medications, supplements, immunizations, diseases, conditions, operations, and symptoms)

❑ Health insurance, Medicare, or Medicaid ID card

❑ Photo ID

❑ Copy of your advance directive and DNR (do not resuscitate) if you have them. (See page 80)

❑ Medicine containers and medication dosages

❑ Change of clothing and personal items in case you spend the night

What happens if I don't have health insurance?

❏ If it is a true medical emergency, you will receive necessary stabilizing treatment.

❏ You can be refused care if the staff evaluated you and do not believe you have a medical emergency as noted above.

❏ You can be transferred to another facility when medically appropriate.

TIP: For future emergencies, identify the people in your mobile phone directory whom you want to be notified in case of emergency by including the letters "ICE" in front of their names. Emergency personnel know to look for such an indicator.

WHAT TO EXPECT IN THE INTENSIVE CARE UNIT (ICU)

*Patients in the intensive care unit are there because
they are critically ill, and that is scary enough.
Add to that the stress of the ICU environment,
and you have one huge scary and frightening experience
for the patient and the family.*

Patient-to-nurse ratio: The ICU patient-to-nurse ratio is usually 2:1, which means that there is usually one nurse caring for two patients. Although this may sound like a small workload for the nurse, it can be quite overwhelming when caring for two critically ill individuals who require intensive care. Be mindful of that.

Infection control:

❑ Wash or foam your hands when you enter and when you leave the room for any reason, to prevent the spread of infection.

❑ Make sure that everyone who enters the room or touches the patient washes or foams, including the staff and visitors.

❑ Wear gowns, masks, gloves, and other protective equipment as directed by the nurse to prevent the spread of infection. When finished with such items, be sure to dispose of them as directed.

❑ *Do not* visit if you are feeling sick.

❑ *Do not* bring live plants or flowers into the ICU.

Communicating with the staff:

❑ Bring pen and notebook with you so you can write down all of your questions and the answers to those questions as needed.

❑ Ask staff members to talk in language you can understand, to spell words you don't understand, to draw diagrams when you need more clarification, and to give you written information as necessary.

❑ Select one person to act as family spokesperson and be the liaison between the staff and the rest of the family.

❑ Be aware that during shift changes, team reporting, and unit emergencies, the nurse may be unavailable for routine nonemergency care or concerns.

❑ Be respectful of ICU quiet times.

❑ Be respectful of the privacy of all patients.

❑ Find out when medical staff rounds are held, and try to be there. Bring your notebook with your written questions, and be sure to get them answered.

When to call the nurse:

❑ The alarm goes off on any equipment being used for patient care

❑ You see blood or other bodily fluids where they aren't supposed to be

❑ A tube becomes disconnected or dislodged

❑ You notice a change in the patient's color, movement, condition, or behavior

❑ You notice an empty intravenous fluid bag

Visiting in the ICU:

❑ Read the **PatientAction.com** article "How to Be a Good Visitor" before you visit or see the worksheet of the same title in this book. (see page 104)

❑ Familiarize yourself with the ICU visiting policy and be mindful of it.

❑ Turn your mobile phone to vibrate. Ask the staff about policies related to its usage in the ICU.

❑ Be careful moving around the room and the patient-care area so you do not knock anything over, pull a tube out, or interfere with the normal functioning of any machines.

❑ Let the nurse know when you leave the patient unit and how you can be contacted if needed.

❑ Provide quiet music that the patient enjoys to promote relaxation.

❑ Speak quietly to the patient even if she or he is not responsive.

❑ Pray quietly with or for the patient.

❑ Read a favorite book or poetry to the patient.

❑ Speak to the nurse about arranging for a clergy visit.

❑ Make eye contact with the patient when communicating.

❑ Do *not* give the patient anything to eat or drink without checking with the nurse.

❑ Hold the patient's hand, rub the arms or legs, give a back rub to reduce stress.

Spending the night in the ICU:

❑ Find out the policy about spending the night from the nurse or nurse manager.

❑ Ask for a pillow, sheets, blanket, and other items you might need if you spend the night.

❑ If you spend the night with the patient, don't expect to have a good night's sleep—you will be disturbed regularly as the staff provide care to the person you are advocating for.

NAVIGATING THE EMERGENCY ROOM (ER) EXPERIENCE

The ER is a scary and stressful place.
Unless you present with a true medical emergency,
the wait to be seen by a doctor can be long and frustrating.
Be prepared for the experience.

What constitutes a medical emergency?
If you have any of the following symptoms, call 911.

❑ Chest pain, suspected heart attack

❑ Poisoning (after you've called the Poison Hotline at
    1- 800-222-1222)

❑ Severe shortness of breath

❑ Uncontrolled or severe bleeding

❑ Suspected overdose of medication

❑ Severe burns

❑ High fever (especially in infants)

❑ Loss of consciousness

❑ Seizures

❑ Diabetic complications such as insulin shock or ketoacidosis

❑ Gunshot or stab wounds

❑ Severe and persistent abdominal pain

Where you can obtain emergency treatment:

❑ Urgent care center—generally open 365 days per year from 8:00 a.m. to 8:00 p.m.

❑ Hospital emergency room—open everyday around the clock

What to bring:

❑ A trusted family member or friend who will act as your Patient Advocate ... or have one meet you there. Allow them to speak for you as needed.

❑ Completed health history (including allergies, medications, supplements, immunizations, disease, conditions, operations, and symptoms).

❑ Health insurance, Medicaid, or Medicare ID card, and photo ID

❑ Pencil and paper for taking notes or writing down questions

❑ Containers from any prescription and/or nonprescription, herbal, supplemental, and over-the-counter drugs you take along with the dosage of each drug or a list of the those drugs.

❑ Advance directive and DNR (do not resuscitate) (See page 80)

❑ A small bag with personal/toiletry items in case you spend the night

❑ Eyeglasses and case

❑ Contact lens case (better to leave contact lenses home)

❑ Next-of-kin contact information

<u>Leave all valuables at home.</u> Don't pack cash or jewelry. Leave your wallet, credit cards, and checkbook home. You will not need them, and there is always a chance that they could disappear.

If you come in with a true medical emergency, you will probably be seen by the doctor immediately. If you come in with a non-medical emergency, you will be assessed by a nurse, who will determine in what order you will be seen by the doctor. Be familiar with the coverage of your health insurance policy. It may not cover you for nonemergency ER care.

What to expect and do upon arrival for a non-emergency:

❑ You will be evaluated by a nurse, who will determine the order in which you will be seen.

❑ Be sure to let the nurse know that you have a patient advocate with you.

❑ Unless you have a true medical emergency, you will probably be seated in the waiting area until it is your turn to be evaluated by the doctor. If the ER is very busy, be prepared to wait for several hours. If you are unable to sit for any reason, ask the nurse if there is a quiet place where you can lie down while waiting.

❑ Be sure to check in with the nurse if you leave the area for any reason.

❑ **Do not** eat or drink anything without speaking with the nurse first.

❑ **Do not** go to the bathroom without asking the nurse if a urine or stool sample will be needed.

❑ **Do not** take any of your own medication without speaking with the nurse first.

What you can do to speed up the process:

❑ Stay calm and pleasant, but be assertive.

❑ If the person you are advocating for or the person advocating for you does not speak English, ask for an interpreter. If no interpreter is available, ask the nurse for the hospital's code for AT&T's 24/7 hotline language service which can be accessed by calling 1-800-752-6096.

❑ Provide staff with your health history (include allergies, medications, immunizations, diseases, conditions, operations, and symptoms).

❑ Provide staff with all the personal information they ask for.

❑ Share all of your symptoms and pertinent health information with the staff.

❑ Let the nurse know if your symptoms change while you are waiting to be seen.

❑ If you've been waiting for a long time, periodically let the staff know that you are still waiting.

Once you are taken into an examination room:

❑ Make sure that *everyone* who touches you or your personal care items has washed their hands.

❑ Use disinfectants to wipe down bed side rails, bedside table, telephone, and nurse call bell.

❑ Ask the staff to disinfect all patient-care equipment such as stethoscopes, scissors, etc., before they use it on you.

❑ Make sure each staff person asks you for your name and/or checks your ID bracelet before administering medication or treatments to you, to prevent any mistakes.

❑ Ask each staff person or anyone you don't recognize, who enters your room his or her name and title, and what role he or she plays in your overall care.

❑ Be aware that you may not be able to use your cell phone and there may be no land line telephone to use.

❑ Write down your questions and be sure you or your advocate ask them so that everyone understands what's going on.

❑ Expect to have your needs met and to be treated with kindness and dignity. If that doesn't happen, report that to the ER nurse manager.

❑ Ask for a clergy visit as necessary.

❑ Be assertive and speak up. **YOU HAVE A VOICE. ... USE IT!**

Diagnostic tests or procedures in the ER:

❑ Ask what the test or procedure is for and what they hope to find out.

❑ Ask if you will have any pain during the test and if you will be given medication for the pain.

❑ Ask who will be doing the test and about the competency of that person.

❑ Ask how and when you will get the results of the test.

❑ Be sure to acquire the written report of the test results.

The role of your patient advocate:

❑ Be with you, support you, and speak for you when you can't speak for yourself

❑ Spend the night with you if necessary

❏ Be sure the hospital and each doctor on your medical team accepts your insurance.

❏ Ask the name and role of every person who gives you care.

❏ Ask the questions you may not think to ask when you are stressed, scared, in pain, or otherwise unable to use your voice.

❏ Help you recall answers to questions that have already been asked

❏ Review consents for treatment with you

❏ Know what medications are being given and why, know what side effects to look for.

❏ Keep in touch with family members and friends regarding your condition.

❏ Make sure that *everyone* who touches you or your personal-care items has washed their hands and disinfected all patient-care equipment.

❏ Ask nurse for disinfectant in order to frequently disinfect bed side rails, bedside table, telephone, TV remote, and nurse call bell.

After being seen in the ER, you will be either held overnight for observation, sent for emergency surgery, admitted to the hospital for further care, transferred to another facility, or sent home. If you are on Medicare, be aware that unless you are actually admitted to the hospital, Medicare may not cover the expenses for you being held in an observational unit. Discuss this with your doctor before she or he sends you to an observation unit without admitting you. *Be sure you understand all of your discharge instructions.* Retain them for follow-up medical appointments.

DIAGNOSTIC TESTING AND PROCEDURES

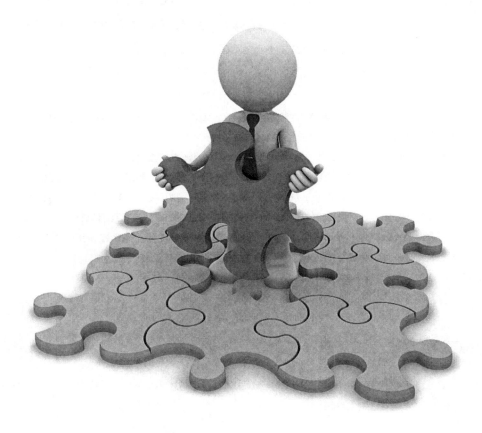

HOW YOUR DIAGNOSIS IS MADE

I talked about my symptoms. The doctor examined me and is now ordering lots of tests. Why do I need them? What do I need to know?

Diagnostic testing is usually required to make a definitive identification of your medical problem (diagnosis) and to determine the best treatment plan. In an attempt to identify your medical problem, your doctor may order a variety of blood tests, diagnostic tests, or procedures. At times, your doctor may also refer you to other health care professionals for assistance in the identification or treatment of that diagnosis. Feel comfortable in telling your doctor that you would like a second opinion once the diagnosis has been made. That is not unusual, and most health insurance companies will reimburse for second opinions.

Preparing for the physical exam:

❑ Bring a patient advocate with you, if possible, and allow him or her to speak for you as needed.

❑ Follow your doctor's instructions in preparation for the physical examination or diagnostic procedure or test.

❑ Bring your completed health history (include allergies, medications, supplements, immunizations, diseases, conditions, operations, and symptoms).

❑ Bring all medicine containers and the doses of those medications, including herbs, supplements, and over-the-counter drugs, or a written list of same.

❑ Bring your health insurance, Medicare, or Medicaid ID card.

❑ Bring paper and pencil so you can write down any information you are given.

❑ Ask for explanations, drawings, spellings, photos, and/or computer handouts of things you don't understand.

❑ Follow all medical directions in preparation for the visit.

❑ Bring a list of your current symptoms.

❑ Bring a written list of questions you might have.

❑ Review the worksheet "Questions to Ask before a Diagnostic Procedure" to find the specific questions you should ask before giving consent for a diagnostic procedure or test. (See page 19)

The three most important questions to ask before giving consent for a diagnostic procedure or test:

❑ What is my main medical problem?

❑ What is the procedure being done?

❑ Why is it important to do this procedure?

Questions to ask after the procedure or test is completed:

❑ When will I get the results?

❑ How do I get written copies of the test results?

❑ If the information doesn't confirm the suspected diagnosis, what is the next step?

❑ What happens if the test results are not normal?

❏ If you are not happy with the results, diagnosis, or treatment plan, get a second opinion.

❏ Research the credentials of any specialist your doctor refers you to at HealthGrades.com. Be sure they accept your insurance.

QUESTIONS TO ASK
BEFORE A DIAGNOSTIC PROCEDURE

Sure, you have confidence in your doctor. But what about all those tests you are being scheduled for?

Try to have the conversation about the diagnostic procedure with your health care provider when you are dressed. The literature shows that patients miss 30% of the information given to them while they are undressed. Be sure to have your patient advocate with you during the conversation.

Why ask the questions?

❑ To be an informed patient

❑ To understand what's happening to you

❑ To be in control of what's going on

❑ To be part of the decision-making process

The questions to ask:

❑ What is my main medical problem?

❑ Why is it important to do this procedure?

❑ How will the procedure be performed?

❑ Where will the procedure be performed?

❑ Is the diagnostic facility in my health insurance network?

❑ Who performs the procedure? Is this practitioner in my health insurance network?

❑ How competent is the person performing the procedure?

❑ What do I need to do to prepare for the procedure?

❑ Are there any risks involved?

❑ Are the benefits worth the risks?

❑ Will it require hospitalization? For how long?

❑ How long will the procedure take?

❑ Do I need someone to accompany me?

❑ How will my anxiety be dealt with?

❑ Will the procedure result in any discomfort, pain, or loss of bodily function? If so, for how long?

❑ How will any discomfort or pain be dealt with?

❑ Will my health insurance company cover the cost?

❑ How and when will I find out the results of the procedure?

❑ Who will be giving me the results?

❑ What happens if the results are not normal?

❑ How do I get a written copy of the results?

❑ Is there a less expensive or less intrusive or invasive procedure that can give the same results?

❑ If the information doesn't confirm the suspected diagnosis, what is the next step?

SO YOU'RE HAVING A COLONOSCOPY

The worst part about having a colonoscopy is the preparation you need to do the day before. The procedure itself is a breeze, thanks to the great drugs they use! Empower yourself to make it a good experience!

Ten days before the test:

❏ Your doctor will send you instructions about your test. Arrange your schedule so you will be at home at the time your preparation for the procedure begins.

❏ Fill the pharmaceutical prescription(s) required for your preparation medication. **Read the instructions** so you have time to seek guidance from the pharmacist if necessary.

❏ Review the doctor's instructions regarding what you can drink or eat during your preparation, and have those items available. If you have any questions, call your doctor. Flavoring your preparation with yellow powdered Crystal Light/Kool-Aid will make it taste better. Be sure your doctor approves of this.

❏ Review all other instructions, and call the doctor with any questions.

❏ Check to see if your preparation medication will need to be refrigerated.

❏ Review the written information so you know what time you have to show up for your procedure and the location of the procedure. Plan to arrive 1–2 hours before the scheduled appointment time.

❏ Prepare your bathroom with toilet paper, *flushable* wipes, and reading material for preparation day.

❏ Alert all family members to your urgent need for the bathroom on preparation day.

❏ Arrange for someone to drive you to the procedure, to be available during the procedure to act as your advocate and to drive you home.

❏ Discuss with your doctor what medications you are taking, and find out which ones you need to omit in preparation for the procedure and which ones are okay to take the day of the procedure.

❏ Unless otherwise indicated on the preparation bottle, refrigerate your preparation medication after you mix it—it will taste much better! Once mixed, the preparation will have an expiration date—be sure to check it.

❏ Update and print out your completed health history (include allergies, medications, supplements, immunizations, diseases, conditions, operations, and symptoms).

On the day before the procedure (preparation day!):

❏ Follow the prescribed clear liquid diet for the entire day.

❏ Carefully follow the instructions for the intestinal preparation medication. If you are not sufficiently cleaned out, the procedure cannot be performed.

❏ Check to see if your prep needs to be refrigerated.

❏ The preparation medication is very salty. If your doctor has approved, add powdered *yellow* Crystal Light/Kool-Aid to the preparation medication. If the prep can be refrigerated, be sure it is cold before you take it and add some ice chips to make it easier to drink. It will taste much better! Holding your nose while drinking the preparation medication through a straw can also be helpful.

- ❏ Once the preparation begins, stay near a bathroom.

- ❏ For comfort and to avoid anal irritation, clean yourself gently with flushable wipes after each bowel movement. Be sure your wipes are flushable and only flush one wipe at a time to avoid clogging your toilet.

- ❏ Follow your doctor's instructions for when you need to stop taking solid foods and fluids.

- ❏ Take only those evening medications that your doctor has preapproved.

On the morning of the test:

- ❏ Do not eat or drink anything unless you have special instructions from your doctor regarding medication.

- ❏ Take any prescription medications that the doctor *preapproved*.

- ❏ Bring your health history with you.

- ❏ Bring your health insurance, Medicaid, or Medicare card with you.

- ❏ Bring photo ID with you.

- ❏ Leave all valuables at home or give them to your trusted advocate during the procedure.

- ❏ Bring a credit card if you have a co-pay or don't have health insurance.

- ❏ Bring reading glasses, if necessary, for filling out any written forms.

- ❏ Arrive for your test 1–2 hours before the scheduled appointment time.

- ❏ Have someone drive you to the procedure, be available during the procedure to act as your advocate and take you home when the procedure is complete. You will be under the influence of medication administered to you.

What to expect upon arrival for the procedure:

❏ The receptionist will go over the standard preliminary questions and make a copy of your insurance card(s).

❏ You will be asked to sign some paperwork. Read forms carefully before signing. Question anything that is unclear. Review the worksheet "Signing a Treatment Consent Form." (See page 86)

❏ You may be asked if the person accompanying you is your designated patient advocate whom the doctor can share pertinent test information with.

❏ Leave all of your personal items with the person accompanying you.

❏ You will be escorted to the pre-procedure area.

❏ You will be greeted by the nurse who will be caring for you throughout the procedure.

❏ Your nurse will ask you to undress, put on the hospital gown, and get into the bed. If you're cold, ask the nurse for a warm blanket.

❏ An intravenous (IV) infusion may be started in one of your arm veins, through which you will later receive wonderful drugs that will put you into "twilight sleep," making you totally unaware of the procedure. Be aware that you might be dehydrated at this point and they may have to stick you more than once to obtain a good vein.

❏ If you have to go to the bathroom, let the nurse know, and she or he will help you navigate the trip with the IV.

❏ You will probably be seen by the anesthesiologist, who is the medical doctor who will manage your sleep.

When the procedure is over:

❏ Upon waking up, you may still be a bit woozy from the drugs.

❏ Your IV will be removed.

❏ You will be assisted with dressing, if necessary.

❏ You or your advocate will be given written post-procedure instructions.

❏ Your doctor will share preliminary findings with you and your designated patient advocate. The advocate is included in this process as you may not recall the instructions because of the medications they used to put you into "twilight sleep."

❏ You will be escorted to your car by a staff person.

❏ You should go home and sleep off the medication.

❏ Do not drive or use any dangerous equipment.

❏ You may pass some excessive rectal gas (flatus) for the first 24–48 hours. This is perfectly normal, as they inserted gas into your intestines during the procedure.

❏ You should be able to resume all regular activities once the medication is out of your system, usually within 12 hours.

Call your doctor immediately if you experience:

❏ Fever

❏ Chills

❏ Severe abdominal pain

❏ Abdominal drainage

❏ Moderate amount of bleeding in your stool

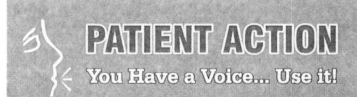

DISEASES/CONDITIONS

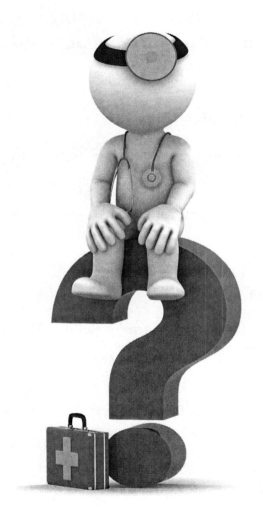

WHEN YOU'RE DIAGNOSED WITH CANCER

Once you've been diagnosed with cancer, you are flooded with emotions of shock, disbelief, and panic. Every ache, every pain, every bump, and every lump makes you worry that your cancer is spreading or coming back. A little knowledge goes a long way in helping you cope with this possibly devastating diagnosis.

When you receive the diagnosis:

❑ Have a trusted patient advocate go with you to every medical appointment.

❑ Empower and encourage your advocate to be an active participant in all discussions.

❑ Bring a pen and notebook to every appointment to record all pertinent information.

❑ Be prepared for every appointment with written questions. Write down the answers.

❑ Ask all members of your health care team to spell words you don't get, to talk in language you can understand, and to draw pictures in your notebook as needed for clarification.

❑ Research your particular cancer on the internet. See below for reliable links and resources.

- ❑ Research online community blogs that address your specific type of cancer.

- ❑ Share all research and/or internet findings with your doctor.

- ❑ Seek out a second opinion (or third) if you feel compelled to do so, but realize that you will ultimately need to put your trust in one doctor.

- ❑ Make sure that the doctor you pick has a passion for your life.

- ❑ Allow loved ones and friends to support you in this journey. Ask for help. Accept help.

- ❑ Don't be afraid to show your emotions. This is scary stuff. If you need to cry, cry, then get on with the business of healing.

- ❑ Reach out to others who have had the same cancer for support through the American Cancer Society or other diagnosis related online blogs.

- ❑ Get professional counseling for yourself and/or family as needed. Seek out the hospital chaplain, regardless of your own faith.

- ❑ Speak to your oncologist about using alternative or complementary forms of treatment along with standard cancer therapy, which usually includes surgery, chemotherapy, radiation therapy, or a combination of one or more. These complementary treatments can include acupuncture, hypnosis, nutrition, visualization, meditation, massage, and more.

- ❑ Speak to your oncologist about clinical trials being done for the cancer you have been diagnosed with. Seek out that information for yourself at the reliable resources listed below.

- ❑ Create a free interactive journal at **www.CaringBridge.com** to keep those who care about you informed about your journey. The personal prayers and inspirational messages they send you will raise your spirits each day.

❑ Have a family member start a **GoFundMe.com** campaign for you to help raise funds to help pay for your medical expenses.

❑ Check out the inspirational sayings and prayers at **www.PatientAction.com** for support and inspiration.

❑ If you are the advocate or caregiver for someone receiving chemotherapy, be sure to take care of yourself, physically and spiritually, so you will be able to cope with your loved one's needs.

There are many places you can go to for information, resources, and assistance. Below is a list of some of these reliable sources:

1. The American Cancer Society, 1-800-227-2345, www.cancer.org

2. Cancer.net

3. Cancer Care, 1-800-813-HOPE (4673), www.cancercare.org

4. Cancer Spiritual Support, www.mystronghold.org

5. Cancer Information Service, 1-800-4-CANCER (1-800-422-6237)

6. www.cancercenter.com, 866-517-8520

7. St Jude's Hospital for childhood cancers, www.stjude.org

8. www.cleaningforareason.org

9. www.voicesagainstbraincancer.org

10. www.stupidcancer.org

11 I Can Cope classes, American Cancer Society, 1-800-227-2345, www.cancer.org

12. Ovarian Cancer Research Fund, www.ocrf.org

13. *What Next?* American Cancer Society, 1-800-227-2345, www.what next.com

14. www.Livestrong.org

15. American Childhood Cancer Organization, 1-855-858-2226, www.acco.org

16. Your local hospital may have a Cancer Hotline.

17. National Cancer Institute/National Institute of Health, www.nci cancergov@mail.nih.gov (for info regarding the most current government research)

18. Sarcoma Foundation of America, 866-501-6780, www.curesar coma.org or info@curesarcoma.org

19. Patient Power (Blood Related Cancers) www.patientpower.info

WHEN YOU NEED CHEMOTHERAPY

You've been diagnosed with cancer and your life has taken a new twist. To regain some control, be sure to ask the right questions so you understand the treatment.

Questions to ask about your chemotherapy treatment:

❑ What type of chemotherapy is most effective for my type of cancer?

❑ What are the chances that this treatment will be effective?

❑ What immediate side effects can I expect from my chemotherapy treatments?

❑ Are any long-term side effects associated with this treatment?

❑ How will the chemotherapy be administered, and by whom?

❑ How often will I need chemotherapy? How long will each individual treatment take?

❑ How many cycles of chemotherapy will I need? (A cycle is a period of time of chemotherapy treatment and recovery before a new dose is given.)

❑ Where will I receive my chemotherapy?

❑ What are the risks associated with this treatment?

❑ How will chemotherapy affect my ability to work or to perform daily tasks?

❑ How will the chemotherapy affect my fertility? (If adolescent or young adult male): Should I save my sperm in a sperm bank? (If childbearing female): Should I save my eggs? How do I go about doing that?

❑ How do I prepare for my chemotherapy?

❑ Will I need to take any precautions during treatment?

❑ How will I know that the chemotherapy is working?

❑ What can I do to maximize the effectiveness of the chemotherapy?

❑ Will I need other treatments besides chemotherapy?

❑ Are there alternative treatments? If so, what are they?

❑ If it doesn't work, what other treatments are available?

❑ Can I refuse treatment?

❑ Are there any complementary treatments I can use during my chemotherapy to help me cope and/or to help maximize the treatments (such as diet, massage, yoga, visualization, meditation, hypnosis, acupuncture)? How do I access them?

HOW DO YOU KNOW IF YOU HAVE AN INFECTION?

Some infections are a nuisance. Others can kill you. Know the symptoms.

A localized infection occurs when an abnormal presence of bacteria, viruses, parasites, or fungi outside the body are causing signs and symptoms. The most common sites of localized infection are the skin and nails.

Signs and symptoms of a localized infection:

❑ Redness at the site

❑ Heat at the site

❑ Swelling at the site

❑ Pain at the site

❑ Yellow pus or other thick drainage from the site

A systemic infection is an abnormal presence of bacteria, viruses, parasites, or fungi in the body that is causing disease. The most common sites of systemic infection are the urinary tract, blood, skin, lungs, and throat.

Signs and symptoms of a systemic infection:

❏ Feeling sick and fatigued

❏ Loss of appetite

❏ Fever

❏ Red streaks on the skin moving away from a localized infection toward the heart

If you suspect you have an infection, seek out medical intervention immediately.

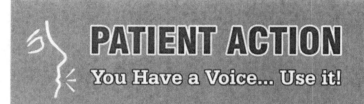

END OF LIFE ISSUES

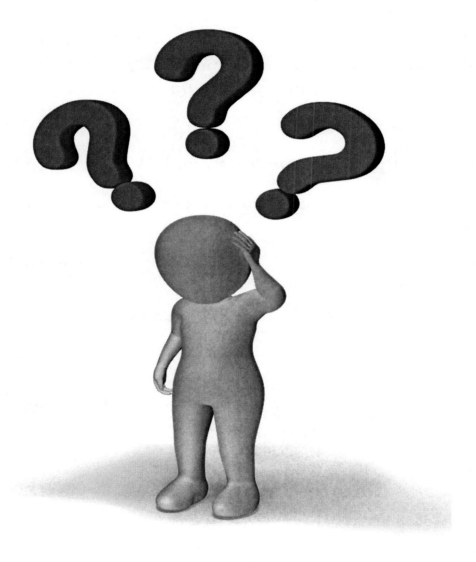

END-OF-LIFE CONVERSATIONS

An end-of-life conversation when the patient is terminally ill could be the hardest conversation you ever have. It could also be the most important. Make it count.

When is the right time for an end-of-life conversation?

❑ The doctor has advised you that the patient is extremely ill with little hope for recovery.

❑ The extremely ill patient indicates that he or she wants to have the conversation.

❑ You feel it is time to have such a conversation with a family member or friend.

How does a family member initiate such a conversation with the terminally ill person?

❑ *"We need to have a difficult conversation."*

❑ *"There are some things we need to talk about that might be uncomfortable."*

❑ *"You're in a rough situation, and I need to explain it to you so you understand what's going on."*

❑ *"Things are not looking good."*

- ❑ *"Things are not going well."*

- ❑ *"Do you want me to be perfectly honest with you?"*

- ❑ *"You need to be part of the decision-making process."*

- ❑ *"There are things I need to share with you."*

- ❑ *"There are things you need to share with me."*

- ❑ *"What do you understand about your illness?"*

- ❑ *"Do you realize that you are not getting better despite maximal medical treatment?"*

Types of Conversations the Dying Person May Want To Have:

- ❑ Sharing and acknowledging thoughts and feelings about family and friends

- ❑ Sharing and acknowledging thoughts and feelings that loved ones may be having

- ❑ Reminiscing about the past

- ❑ Being reassured that they will not suffer

- ❑ Being reassured that they will not die alone

- ❑ Being reassured that their family will be okay upon their death

- ❑ Being reassured that they will be missed

- ❑ Being reassured they have brought value to the lives of loved ones and friends

- ❑ Saying good-bye to loved ones and friends

Reasons why families might avoid this conversation:

❑ It is a hard and painful conversation that forces family members to face their own mortality.

❑ They may feel they lack the right words.

❑ Some people are afraid to talk about death and dying.

❑ The family or patient is often in denial and refuses to acknowledge the end of life.

Ways for family members to communicate that they care:

❑ Offer a visit from the clergy.

❑ Encourage the expression of feelings, and carefully listen to them.

❑ Hold hands, give back rubs, lie in bed with your loved one.

❑ Express your appreciation of the relationship you have shared together.

❑ Express your love.

❑ Express your support and commitment to be with your loved one through this part of his or her final journey.

❑ Encourage your loved one to reminisce about the past.

❑ Tell your loved one that they will be missed.

❑ Recite a prayer with your loved one (several prayers can be found at **PatientAction.com** at the link for **"PRAYERS"**).

❑ Cry with or for your loved one to show your sadness.

❑ Joke or laugh appropriately.

❑ Give your loved one opportunities for making his or her own decisions whenever possible.

❑ Ask your loved one if she or he has any final requests, and have them fulfilled, if possible.

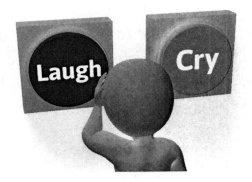

WHEN YOU OR YOUR LOVED ONE NEEDS HOSPICE

Although caring for your terminally ill loved one at home is a very noble and loving gesture, the reality is that even the most well-intentioned families cannot do this on their own. There is help!

A person is considered terminally ill when the personal physician certifies that the life expectancy is less than 6 months, regardless of their current state of health.

Hospice care is an alternative approach for providing care to the terminally-ill or to the patient whose disease is progressing despite maximal treatment.

What is hospice?

❑ Hospice care is an alternative approach for providing care to the terminally-ill patient whose disease is progressing despite maximal treatment.

❑ Hospice also provides palliative care for the management of symptoms associated with any chronic illnesses that the patient may be suffering from, at any stage of their illness.

❑ Hospice is a way of caring, not a specific place.

❑ Hospice care is usually a formal program directed by a physician and administered by a nurse.

❏ Hospice provides care that meets the special needs of terminally ill persons of all ages and their family members.

❏ Hospice helps the patient decide about their own care and how they manage the life they have left, as well as how and where they will die.

❏ Hospice helps the family affirm life, enables the patient to live until he or she dies, and helps the family to live with the patient as they the patient is dying ... and to go on living afterward.

❏ Hospice eases the physical, emotional, and spiritual pain and suffering of the patient and family, and supports the family in the care of their terminally ill loved one.

❏ Hospice is about living. It provides for quality of life, not quantity of days.

Why Hospice?

❏ Caregivers use up all their energy providing the physical and challenging care.

❏ With Hospice doing the physical care, families can spend those last weeks and months sharing happy memories, saying good-bye, and sharing their love.

❏ Families eventually find themselves overwhelmed and unable to cope with the physical strain and the roller-coaster emotions of caring for a terminally ill loved one.

❏ Hospice takes over the job of caregiving so each family member can resume his or her role as loving wife, husband, partner, parent, or child.

How do you know your loved one is ready for hospice?

❑ Does your loved one have a life-limiting diagnosis?

❑ Is your loved one frail, with other progressive medical problems?

❑ Is the disease progressing despite maximal medical treatment?

❑ Does your loved one have frequent hospitalizations, recurring infections, or unscheduled office visits?

❑ Has your loved one's function or nutritional status declined in the past 30 days?

If you answered *yes* to one or more of these questions, it might be time to discuss hospice care with the patient's primary physician.

Where is Hospice?

❑ In the patient's home, wherever that might be (nursing home, rehab facility, assisted living)

❑ In a specialized unit of the hospital

❑ In a free-standing hospice facility

Who makes up the hospice team?

❑ Doctors and nurses

❑ Social workers

❑ Pastoral counselors

❑ Bereavement counselors

❑ Financial and legal counselors

❑ Caretakers

❑ Homemakers

❑ Volunteers who provide respite for the family

Who pays for hospice?

❑ Every patient is accepted into hospice, regardless of ability to pay.

❑ If the hospice program is Medicare-certified, the care will be covered by the Medicare Hospice Benefit.

❑ Hospice is an optional benefit under Medicaid.

❑ Hospice is covered by many private insurance companies. Check your health insurance policy to see if it covers hospice care.

GIVING HOPE TO THE DYING PATIENT

When a person is very ill, hope is a valuable coping tool to promote quality of life and sense of well-being. Be sure you know how to provide that hope to your loved one so your loved one does not feel isolated and abandoned.

How a doctor provides hope to the dying person:

❑ Providing honest assessment of the medical situation.

❑ Letting the patient know he or she is valued.

❑ Treating the entire person physically, spiritually, and psychologically.

❑ Including the person in all decision making.

How you can provide hope to your seriously ill or dying loved one:

❑ Encourage your loved one to talk, and listen to what he or she has to say.

❑ Involve your loved one in all decision making when he or she is able.

❑ Encourage your loved one to be independent.

❑ Never trivialize your loved one's feelings.

❑ Try to honor your loved one's requests.

❑ Tell your loved one how much you value him or her and how much he or she means to you.

❑ Share your own feelings with your loved one.

❑ Help your loved one reminisce about past joyful times.

❑ Look at family memorabilia and photos together.

❑ Sing songs together with your loved one, or sing for him or her.

❑ Provide your loved one with a way to listen to favorite music.

❑ Watch favorite television shows together.

❑ Read together.

❑ Play games together.

❑ Offer to make phone calls or to send e-mails or other notes on your loved one's behalf.

❑ Let your loved one know that she or he will be missed.

❑ Talk about religious beliefs, and offer to have a clergy member visit.

❑ Create a sense of well-being in your loved one's room by being appropriately supportive?

❑ Provide assurance that your loved one will not be alone, that you will be there with him or her.

❑ Hold your loved one's hands, gently rub his or her back, legs, or arms.

❑ Climb into bed with your loved one and cuddle.

❑ Cry with your loved one when appropriate, but be sure to look for opportunities to laugh as well.

❑ Focus on the life of your loved one in the last days and hours.

It is certainly fine to tell your loved one to hope for the best while at the same time preparing for the worst. Discussions about the illness, prognosis, and treatment are appropriate and necessary. Such discussions provide the patient with the opportunity to ask questions, and to seek clarification and understanding.

What do you do if the person refuses to discuss his or her illness, prognosis, or treatment with you?

If the patient refuses to discuss such matters with you or with his or her health care team, it is probably because the person is not yet ready to grapple with the significance of such discussions. The ill family member may very well still be in denial, which is the first stage of grieving, still in the process of mourning for his or her own potential loss of life.

Let the person grieve. Give the person space to mourn. Let their heart take them wherever they need to go at any given time. Let him or her know that you care and that you will be there for them no matter what. Seek out intervention from a professional counselor or therapist as needed to help you or the patient cope.

FINANCES AND HEALTH CARE

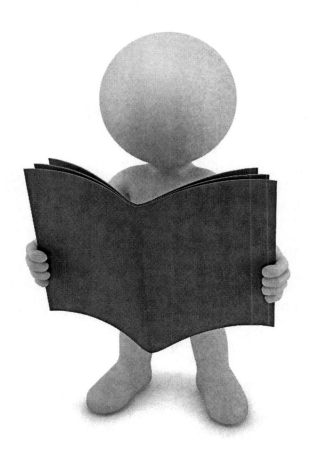

DEALING WITH YOUR
HEALTH INSURANCE COMPANY

*Getting your voice heard by your health insurance
company is often difficult and frustrating.
Learn how to work the system.*

Preparing for the Call:

Expect this phone call to last a while. Prepare *a* list of the questions
you want answered.

❏ Set aside some quiet time and space for making the phone call.

❏ Review your health insurance benefits booklet and have it available.

❏ Be familiar with what co-payments (co-pays) you are required to pay.

❏ Be familiar with any individual/family deductibles you are required
to meet or have already met.

❏ Be familiar with your drug coverage.

❏ Have all relevant bills available.

❏ Have your health insurance ID card available.

❏ Have paper and pencil available.

❏ Take some deep breaths as needed to help you control any stress that
may occur as a result of the call.

Once you are connected on the Call:

❑ Stay calm, focused, and assertive!

❑ Give them your call back phone number in case you get diconnected.

❑ Document the names of all people with whom you speak, the date and the time you spoke with them, their titles, and all relevant information received. Ask for clarification on anything you don't understand. Write it down. If your claim or request is denied, ask to speak with a supervisor, and go up the chain of command until you get satisfaction. When all else fails, speak with the insurance company's doctor who has the ultimate decision regarding your claim, or have your personal doctor speak for you.

Name of insurance rep 1 _____

Title _____   Date & time _____

Relevant information _____

Name of insurance rep 2 _____

Title _____   Date & time _____

Relevant information _____

Name of insurance rep 3 _____

Title _____   Date & time _____

Relevant information _____

Name of insurance company physician _____

Direct telephone number _____

Best day & time to contact _____

HOW YOUR MEDICAL BILLS GET PAID

The bottom line is that you are required to pay for your medical bills. The bills will not go away.

The Health Care Facility Responsibility:

❑ The hospital staff will do whatever it can to help you pay your hospital bills.

❑ The hospital will file claims for you with your health care insurer or other programs such as Medicare or Medicaid.

❑ The hospital will help your doctor with necessary documentation needed to process your bills.

❑ The hospital will help you make arrangements to help you pay for your care.

❑ The hospital will help you set up a payment plan if you do not have health coverage.

Your Health Care Provider's Responsibility:

❑ Your health care provider will do whatever he or she can to help you pay your bills.

❑ Your health care provider will file claims for you with your health care insurer or other programs such as Medicare or Medicaid.

❏ Your health care provider will provide the necessary documentation needed to process your bills.

❏ Your health care provider will help you make arrangements to help you pay for your care.

Your Financial Responsibility:

❏ You need to do whatever you can to pay your hospital bills.

❏ Be sure to request an itemized statement of all medical/hospital bills so you are familiar with what the bills are.

❏ Write down all of your questions before making the phone calls and be prepared to write down all of the answers you get.

❏ Contact your health care provider or hospital's billing office for any questions you might have regarding your bill.

❏ Write down the date, time and name(s) of all person's you speak to and their responses to your questions.

❏ Be sure to let them know if you have no insurance.

❏ Be sure to ask them if all of your treatment codes have been correctly processed.

❏ Contact your health care insurers or the health benefits manager at your place of employment for any questions regarding the benefits you're covered for under your health care insurance.

❏ Provide all of the essential information necessary to the appropriate parties in order to help you get your bills paid.

❏ Be firm with what you can afford to pay.

❏ Negotiate with your health care provider or your hospital's billing department to see if they can reduce your bill.

❑ Work with your health care provider or hospital to see if they will accept low monthly payments until your bill is paid off.

❑ Be patient, be cooperative, be pleasant, be humble, be non-threatening.

❑ If all else fails, make an appointment to speak with the department supervisor face to face. Dress nicely. Be polite. Speak from your heart.

❑ Have a family member start a **GoFundMe.com** campaign for you to raise money and pay for medical expenses.

Be assured that no one can take your home away if you default on medical payments. But they can put a lien on it. And they can destroy your credit rating. Consider your health care provider and hospital as a friend, not an enemy. Health care costs are high. Somebody has to pay for them.

HEALTH CARE SETTINGS

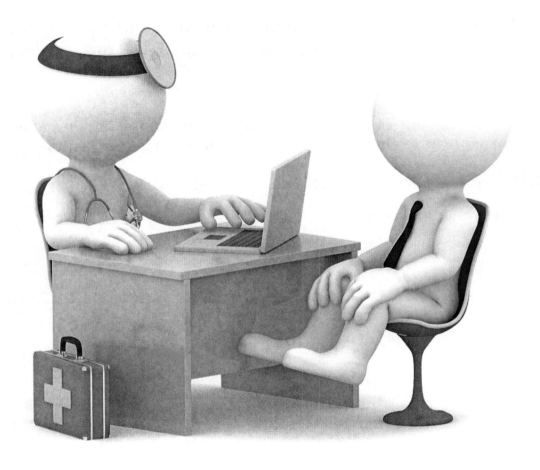

HOW TO SELECT A REHABILITATION, NURSING OR LONG TERM CARE FACILITY

You need to do some research when you want the very best long-term care for you or your loved one.

*This worksheet can also be used when researching nursing homes, assisted-living, rehabilitation and other long-term care facilities.

Make a list of potential facilities in your area:

Name & address of facility 1 _____

_____

_____

Contact person _____

Phone number _____

Time & date of appointment _____

Name & address of facility 2 _____

_____

_____

Contact person _____

Phone number _____

Time & date of appointment _____

Name & address of facility 3 _____

_____

_____

Contact person _____

Phone number _____

Time & date of appointment _____

**Check out the facility at HealthGrades.com,
QualityCheck.org, or HospitalCompare.hhs.gov.**

Things to consider when visiting the facility:

❏ Is the facility licensed and accredited?

❏ How many registered nurses (RNs) and licensed practical nurses (LPNs) are on staff?

❏ What is the staff-to-resident ratio on each shift?

❏ What kind of security is maintained to protect the residents?

❏ Are background checks and random drug testing done on staff?

❏ What therapies are offered, and how often are they available? (Therapies can include speech, physical, and occupational therapies.)

❏ What is the level of family involvement in any therapies offered at the facility?

❏ Ask to see the monthly calendar of activities.

❏ Ask to see the monthly menu calendar from the dietitian. What is served, and what are the second choices? Will they accommodate your or your loved one's personal diet?

❏ Ask about family involvement in the general care of the residents.

❏ Is there an in-house doctor? Can patients use their own personal doctors?

❏ Do the residents look comfortable and well cared for? Are their nails clean? Are they dressed? Is their hair well groomed? Are the men shaved?

❏ Do the staff members look happy and calm?

❏ Do the staff members interact well with the residents and with each other?

❏ Does the facility offer on-site haircuts?

❏ Does the facility offer on-site podiatry nail care?

❏ Does the facility offer TV for each patient?

❏ Will your loved one have a bedside telephone? If not, provide your loved one with a simple cell phone.

❏ Is the facility sensitive to roommate-incompatibility issues?

❏ What are the visitation rules?

❏ Can the residents leave for outings with family or friends?

❑ Does the facility get outside visits from community volunteer groups, both adults and children?

❑ Does the facility have cats, dogs, or other animals for the enjoyment of the residents? Can residents bring their own pets?

How to ease the transition for your loved one:

❑ Make short frequent visits during the first few days and then establish a convenient visiting schedule. Try to vary your long-term visiting schedule so the staff never know when you might show up.

❑ Call frequently.

❑ Be sure to show up when you say you are going to, or call if you are unable to show up.

❑ Bring items that are personal and meaningful for your loved one.

❑ Tape large photographs of family and friends on your loved one's wall as permitted by the facility.

❑ Keep lines of communication open between you, your loved one, and the staff.

❑ Be honest and compassionate with your loved one.

❑ Encourage your loved one to get involved with the activities in the facility.

❑ Participate in meals and facility activities with your loved one, and encourage other family members and friends to do the same.

WHEN YOU'RE BEING ADMITTED TO THE HOSPITAL

Being admitted to the hospital can be stressful, overwhelming and frightening. This worksheet will help you prepare yourself for your hospitalization.

What to bring with you:

❏ A trusted patient advocate, or have one meet you at the hospital. Allow your advocate to speak for you as needed.

❏ Completed health history (including allergies, medications, supplemets, immunizations, diseases, conditions, operations, and symptoms).

❏ Health insurance ID, Medicare, or Medicaid cards

❏ Photo ID

❏ Personal toiletries

❏ Change of clothing and underwear (loose-fitting clothing if you are having surgery)

❏ Sleepwear

❏ Slippers that are slip-proof and easy to slip on

❏ Flip-flops for the shower

❏ Eyeglasses and eyeglass case

- ❏ Contact lens storage case and cleaning supplies (though it's better to leave contact lenses home and wear eyeglasses)

- ❏ Dentures and storage case (labeled with patient's name)

- ❏ Phone numbers of family and friends

- ❏ Your own pillow with a few brightly colored pillowcases

- ❏ The donation certificate if you have donated your own blood

- ❏ Inexpensive iPod or CD player with earphones for the delightful distraction of music

- ❏ Notebook and writing utensils for writing down all of your questions and other relevant information.

- ❏ All of your medication containers and the dosages you take, including prescription drugs, over-the-counter drugs, herbs, and/or supplements (Be prepared to send them home once your assigned nurse completes your admission assessment.) or a complete and current written list of same.

- ❏ A copy of your health care advance directive, including health care proxy, living will, and DNR (do not resuscitate). If you don't have these documents and desire to obtain them, let your advocate and nurse know. Visit **www.putitinwriting.com** for more information about advanced directives (see page 80)

What to leave at home:

- ❏ Money

- ❏ Wallet/Purse

- ❏ Credit cards

- ❏ All valuables, including jewelry

❑ Contact lenses, if possible (bring eyeglasses)

❑ Expensive clothing and footwear

**Be sure to let your health care team know who
your designated patient advocate is going to be.**

What your advocate will be doing:

❑ Be present during health care team rounds.

❑ Advocate for you regarding treatment options.

❑ Advocate for you regarding your advance directive.

❑ Ask the questions you need asked, and express your concerns.

❑ Explain things to you that need clarification.

❑ Confirm that you are getting the right medications.

❑ Help you with treatment or procedure consent forms.

❑ Help you with medical decisions, or make the decisions for you.

❑ Advocate for your discharge planning.

❑ Spend the night at your bedside, if necessary.

HEALTH CARE TEAM

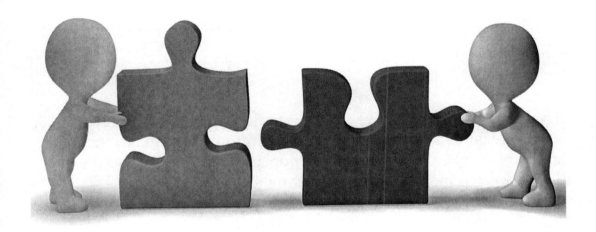

HOW TO PREPARE FOR A DOCTOR VISIT

I always forget to ask my doctor something. This simple checklist will help you prepare for your next doctor visit.

Doctor's name_____

Address_____

Specialty_____

Phone number_____

If possible, do some research on the internet in preparation for your visit so you are familiar with your medical condition. This will facilitate a better discussion between you and your doctor and will give you the benefit of a greater understanding of your medical status.

What to bring with you:

❑ A trusted patient advocate for any appointment other than a wellness visit

❑ Completed health history (including allergies, medications, supplemets, immunizations, diseases, conditions, operations, and symptoms)

❑ All containers of medication and dosage instructions (including non-prescription, herbal, over-the-counter, and supplemental drugs), or a written list of same

- [ ] Your health insurance, Medicare, or Medicaid ID card

- [ ] Copies of any other doctor reports, or lab or diagnostic test results

- [ ] Paper and pencil to write down the information given to you by the health care team

- [ ] Written description of your symptoms

- [ ] Written list of questions (remember that no question is stupid)

- [ ] Credit card, cash, or checkbook to pay your co-pay

Be sure to have been fasting, if necessary, in preparation for any lab tests the doctor will order.

If your doctor prescribes medication for you at the visit, be sure to discuss generic drug options that could save you a lot of money.

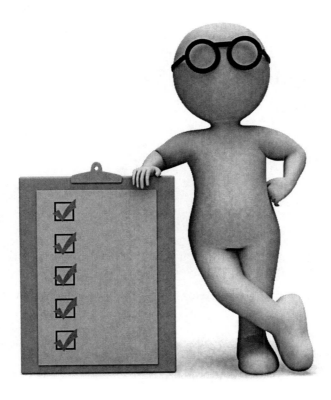

HOW TO SELECT A DOCTOR

You have choices when it comes to doctors. You should feel comfortable with your doctor as a person and confident in his or /her abilities. This is a list of questions to help you determine if the doctor you are thinking of visiting is the right doctor for you. Keep in mind that sometimes you have to forgo the warm and fuzzy heart for the expert brain when you require the services of a medical specialist.

Research your prospective doctor's credentials at HealthGrades.com.

Questions to ask yourself when interviewing a prospective doctor:

❑ Do you feel comfortable with the doctor?

❑ Does the doctor make eye contact with you?

❑ Does the doctor listen to what you have to say?

❑ Does the doctor appear to be interested in your life?

❑ Does the doctor answer your questions respectfully and completely?

❑ Does the doctor spend adequate time with you?

Other important information to consider in your selection process:

❑ Is the doctor in your health insurance network?

❑ Are the office hours convenient for you and your family?

❑ Does the office call back system work for you?

❑ How long does it take to get a call back from the doctor or nurse?

❑ How many other doctors are in the practice?

❑ What is the availability of night calls?

❑ Are there nurse practitioners or physician assistants in the practice? When might you see them instead of the doctor? Can you refuse to see them?

❑ Can you communicate with your doctor by fax or e-mail? What is the turn around time for a response?

❑ Does your doctor practice at a hospital convenient for you? If so, is this hospital in your health insurance network?

❑ How long is the usual wait in the doctor's waiting room? Can you call ahead of time to find out the wait?

❑ What is the average wait once you are taken into an examination room?

❑ How much time does the doctor spend with the average patient?

❑ Is your doctor licensed to practice medicine in the state he is practicing in?

❑ Is your doctor board-certified in his or her specialty?

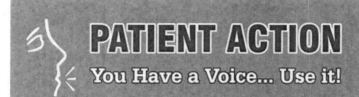

HEALTHY LIVING

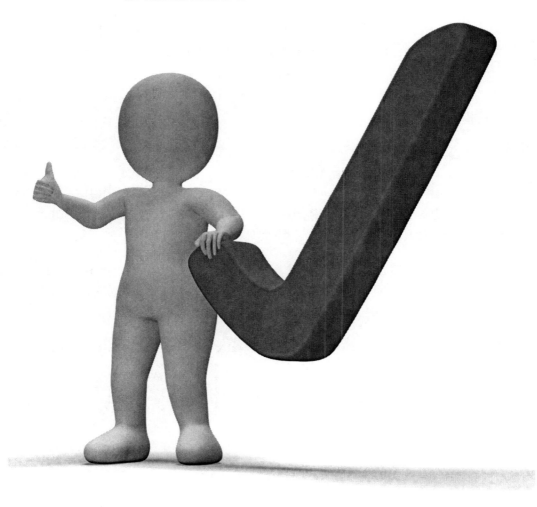

TIPS FOR KEEPING YOUR FAMILY HEALTHY

Raising a healthy family is a huge responsibility, and it isn't an easy task. Learn how to keep your family safe and healthy.

Hand hygiene:

❑ Perform effective hand washing regularly, especially when coming in from outside, before eating, after using the bathroom, after blowing your nose, and whenever else appropriate.

❑ Hum or sing the ABCs or the "Happy Birthday" song while washing your hands with soap and warm water to be sure you're washing for the proper length of time (30 seconds).

❑ Use clean paper towel or tissue to turn off faucets in bathrooms and to open doors of public bathrooms.

❑ Carry and use sanitizing hand cleaner as needed.

Miscellaneous infection control:

❑ Bring sanitizing spray with you during hotel stays and sanitize light switches, remote controls, door knobs, telephones, toilet flusher and seat, faucets, showers, bathtubs, etc.

❑ Place hotel TV remote control inside a ziplock bag.

❑ Use the sanitizing wipes supplied in the grocery store to wipe down the shopping cart handle and the area where babies are placed.

❑ Gargle with an antiseptic mouthwash twice each day if you feel like you are getting a cold or the flu or if you have been exposed to a person suffering with a cold or the flu.

❑ Don't allow anyone with cold- or flu-like symptoms into your home.

❑ Be sure that all who come into your home from the outside wash or sanitize their hands.

❑ Have people remove their shoes before they enter your home.

❑ Keep bottles of hand sanitizer in your car, on your kitchen counter, and in other strategic places in your home and at work.

❑ Avoid biting your nails, as germs accumulate under the nails.

❑ Dispose of dirty tissues immediately to prevent exposure to germs.

❑ Stay home and rest when you suspect you are getting sick.

❑ Keep current with immunizations.

❑ Cover your mouth with a tissue when coughing or sneezing, or cough or sneeze into the elbow joint.

❑ Do not eat or drink from someone else's plate or cup and do not share eating utensils.

❑ Wear socks with your shoes to avoid foot sweating and the risk of fungal infections.

❑ Wear inexpensive flip-flops in public and hotel showers to avoid foot infections.

❑ Avoid walking barefoot outside. If you should sustain a puncture wound or animal bite, go directly to your family doctor or local emergency room.

❑ Keep your hands away from your mouth and face, as your hands harbor disease-causing organisms.

❑ If you have toddlers, sanitize toys regularly with a nontoxic "green" product.

❑ Prepare a 1:10 household mixture of bleach and water to be used for disinfection around your house, but don't use it on fabric or carpet that can be damaged by bleaching.

Infection control in the kitchen:

❑ Do not allow anyone to place their handbag, backpack, briefcase, or similar item on food-prep areas.

❑ Follow food preparation, storage, and refrigeration instructions printed on food labels.

❑ Wash kitchen items including cutting boards used to prepare raw fish, meat, or poultry with hot soap and water before reusing.

❑ Disinfect kitchen sponges by soaking in a bleach solution, "zapping" them in the microwave, or running them through your dishwasher on the sanitizing cycle once a week. Ideally, replace sponges every month.

❑ Disinfect kitchen counters weekly or more often as needed.

❑ Wash all raw fruits and vegetables carefully before eating them.

❑ Peel fruits before eating or buy organic if you are concerned about being exposed to pesticides.

Infection control in nail salons:

❑ Be sure that all nail tools are properly sanitized or bring your own.

❑ Ask them to properly sanitize the foot spa while you watch.

❑ Avoid acrylic or gel nails that can increase the risk for fungal infections.

Female issues:

❑ Reduce risk of vaginal infection by wearing cotton underwear, avoiding spas and bubble baths, and not sitting around in a moist or wet bathing suit.

❑ Schedule annual visits to the gynecologist for early detection of women's health issues.

❑ Participate in safe sex, using condoms to prevent infections.

❑ Perform breast self-examination (BSE) monthly to detect for any lumps or changes in the tissue.

❑ If you are 40 years or older or have a family history of breast cancer, discuss an annual mammogram with your primary doctor.

Male issues:

❑ If you are 18 years or older, examine your testicles monthly to detect for any lumps or changes in the tissue.

❑ Participate in safe sex, using condoms to prevent infections.

❑ If you are 40 years or older or have a family history of prostate cancer, discuss a Protein Specific Antigen (PSA) blood test with your primary doctor.

Healthy living:

❑ Eat a balanced diet with an emphasis on whole grains, fish, fruits, and vegetables.

❑ Get an adequate amount of sleep each night. The average adult requires at least 7–8 hours; elementary school-age children require 10–11 hours; middle school-age children require 9–10 hours; and high school students require 8–9 hours.

❑ Talk to your doctor about how much water you should drink each day.

❑ Quit smoking to dramatically reduce the risk of disease.

❑ Quit chewing tobacco to reduce your risk of oral cancer.

❑ Ensure that you and your family have dental checkups at least once each year. Be sure the dentist checks for oral cancers

❑ Use dental floss once a day to remove plaque and minimize risk of gum infection or disease.

❑ If you are over 50 years of age or have a family history of colon cancer, speak with your family doctor about having a colonoscopy.

❑ Ensure that you and your family have annual wellness examinations.

❑ Exercise for 30 minutes at least 3 times per week.

❑ Avoid caffeine, which is a stimulant and increases stomach acid production.

❑ Avoid drinking diet soda, which increases your risk for pancreatic cancer and other organ disease.

❑ Identify the stressors in your life and figure out what helps you relieve them.

❑ Make time for individual and family recreation to promote family bonding and emotional health.

❑ Plan family dinner time at least twice a week to promote family bonding and communication. Children have voices; let them use those voices, and listen carefully to what they have to say.

❑ Switch household cleaning substances to "green" products to promote a healthier family and world.

❑ Ensure that family members do not share face, hand, or bath towels.

❑ Ensure that family members do not share toothbrushes or bathroom cups.

Listen to your body.
You know it best.
Pursue medical intervention when things
don't seem or feel right.

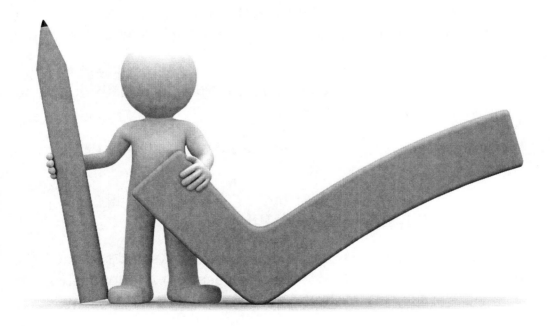

TIPS FOR KEEPING YOUR FAMILY HEALTHY WHEN TRAVELING

Not every location that you might visit has the same standards of sanitation that you are accustomed to. Learn how to keep your family safe and healthy while traveling.

Hand Hygiene:

❏ Perform effective hand washing on a regular basis, especially when coming in from the outside, before eating, after using the bathroom, after blowing your nose, and whenever else appropriate.

❏ Hum or sing the ABC's or Happy Birthday song while washing your hands with soap and warm water to be sure you're washing for the proper length of time (30 seconds).

❏ Use clean paper towel or tissue to turn off faucets in bathrooms and to open doors of public bathrooms.

❏ Carry & use sanitizing hand cleaner as needed.

Miscellaneous infection control:

❏ Bring sanitizing spray with you during hotel stays and sanitize light switches, remote controls, door knobs, telephones, toilet flusher and seat, faucets, showers, bathtubs, etc.

❑ Place hotel TV remote controls inside a ziplock bag.

❑ Do not put your luggage on the hotel beds or luggage racks until you check the beds and nearby end tables and luggage racks for bed bugs. Place your luggage in the bathtub while you check along the edging of the mattresses, linens, the drawers of nearby furniture, and under the straps of luggage racks. If you find even one bug, demand a new room. If 2+ rooms have bed bugs, run from the facility as fast as you can!

❑ Keep a bottle of hand sanitizer in your car, travel bag, back pack, purse.

❑ If you are traveling out of your home country, check the government's Center For Disease Control at **www.CDC.gov** for special alerts and precautions you should take for countries with high risk of infectious diseases and other unsafe conditions.

❑ If you are traveling to a tropical or high temperature location, be sure to bring lots of suntan lotion with you, no less than Broad Spectrum SPF 30 protection. Be sure to also bring sunglasses, protective clothing as needed, and sun hats.

❑ If you are traveling to a country that is at risk for the newly identified Zika virus, be sure to bring an EPA registered insect repellants with DEET, pircaridin, oil of lemon eucalyptus (OLE) or IR 3535.

❑ Men and women traveling to high risk areas for the Zika virus should be sure to have safe and protected anal, vaginal and/or oral sex to avoid getting the Zika virus through sexual contact.

❑ Stay in and rest if you feel like you are getting sick.

❑ Keep current with immunizations for the whole family and bring the immunization records with you to foreign countries.

❑ Be sure to protect your passport when traveling. Consider making a photocopy of the page with your photo and number on it so you can reference it in case you lose your passport while traveling. You do not have to keep your passport with you at all times when you are sight-seeing in other countries unless you will be traveling between countries or a tour guide tells you to bring it. Lock it up in the hotel safe when sightseeing. Do keep the photocopy with you...just in case.

❑ Travel with photocopies of the front and back of all credit cards and other important cards you carry in your wallet in case you lose your wallet. Obviously, do not carry these photocopies in your wallet!

❑ If you are traveling with a child who is not your biological child, be sure to have the proper legal documentation with you to enable you to travel outside of the homeland with that child and to make any necessary medical decisions on that child's behalf should a medical emergency arise while you are traveling.

❑ No matter where you travel, keep your children close by and visible to you at all times.

❑ Wear flip flops in public and hotel showers to avoid foot infections.

❑ Avoid walking barefoot outside where you can pick up organisms or sustain a puncture wound.

❑ If you should sustain a puncture wound or animal bite go directly to the nearest emergency facility for treatment and a possible tetanus shot.

❑ If you are traveling to a remote or dangerous location outside of your homeland, be sure to register with the local American Embassy so that they know you are in the country.

LEGAL DOCUMENTS

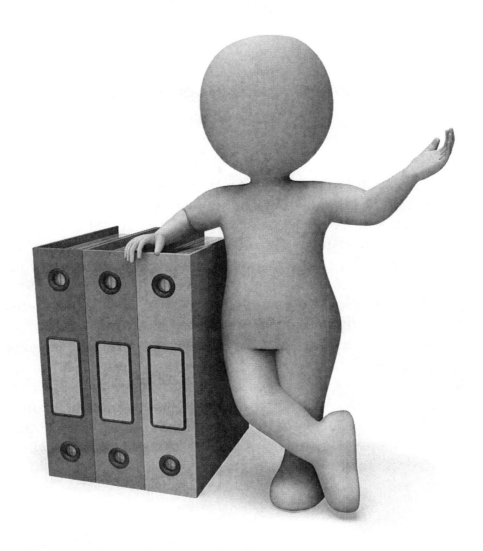

WHAT YOU NEED TO KNOW ABOUT ADVANCE DIRECTIVES

Make the decisions now that you may not be able to make later.

No matter how painful they may be, it is important to have end-of-life conversations with your family while you are healthy. It is never too early to make decisions about the medical care you would want or don't want if you became unable to use your voice to direct your own care. Have you thought about who you would trust as your advocate to make medical decisions for you if you were unable to do so yourself? Have you decided about the withholding or withdrawal of life-sustaining procedures and/or treatment of a terminal condition with no hope for your physical recovery? Advance directives are legal documents that include a health care proxy, durable power of attorney, and living will. Additional documents, including DNRs (do not resuscitate) and, in some states, MOSTs (medical orders for scope of treatment) are also available. An advance directive gives you the opportunity to direct your own care in the event that you are unable to use your voice for any reason. It also provides a means of making financial decisions when you are unable to do so for yourself.

Things to do when planning for an advance directive:

❑ Discuss your advance directive decisions with your family.

❑ Seek the assistance of your personal attorney to complete and file your advance directive.

- ❑ Provide your family with a copy of your advance directive.

- ❑ Be sure that all original documents are notarized by a notary public in your state, if applicable.

- ❑ Keep your original advance directive in a safe and easily accessible place (locked fireproof safety box, not a bank vault). Be sure your family has access to the box.

- ❑ Provide each one of the physicians you see regularly with a copy of your advance directive to file as part of your permanent medical record.

- ❑ If you do not have an advance directive, speak with your attorney; if you are hospitalized and have not yet signed an advance directives, let your nurse know you wish to create one.

- ❑ Keep a small wallet card on your person with the contact information for your health care proxy and alternate and for your durable power of attorney and alternate in the event that you are unable to provide that information when the health care team might need it. You can also add the letters "ICE" (in case of emergency) in front of their first names in your cell phone contact list so medical personnel can iden- tify them when you are unable to do so.

- ❑ If you move to another state, be aware that advance directives vary from state to state. Seek the advice of a local attorney for such pur- pose if you move.

- ❑ Many states offer you the opportunity to register your advance direc- tive in a secure data based computer system for such purpose. There is a small fee for each form registered, but it offers easy access to heath care providers and facilities as needed.

Identification of your health care proxy:

Ask a trusted family member or friend to be your health care proxy. This person will make medical decisions for you when you cannot make them for yourself, such as when you are asleep during surgery or other procedure. Be sure to name an alternate proxy in case the primary one is unable to perform the role at your time of need.

Name of advocate _____

Relationship _____

Telephone number (h)_____ (m) _____

Alternate advocate _____

Relationship _____

Telephone number (h)_____ (m) _____

Identification of your durable power of attorney:

Your durable power of attorney (DPOA) will be the person you designate to make financial decisions for you when you are unable to make them for yourself. Be sure to ask a trusted family member or friend to be your DPOA. Designate a second person to watch over the first designee. Be careful whom you choose. Your DPOA may need to be registered with your state. Discuss this with your personal attorney.

Name of DPOA _____

Relationship _____

Telephone number (h)_____ (m) _____

Alternate DPOA _____

Relationship _____

Telephone number (h)_____ (m) _____

Living will:

This document deals with the end-of-life decisions that arise when your condition is terminal and incurable. It gives you the power to direct your own care when you cannot use your own voice. Share your desires for such care with your family while you are healthy so everyone knows your wishes. Discuss this with your personal attorney.

Visit **www.putitinwriting.org** for more detailed information about Advance Directives.

HOW TO ACCESS YOUR MEDICAL RECORDS

Your medical records belong to you and you have a right to see them or have a copy of them. Accessing them is not always an easy process! Provide as much advance time as possible when requesting records.

To obtain copies of your medical records directly from your physician:

Keep a list of all physicians you have seen in order to make accessing any of your medical records from these physicians easier to obtain when needed.

Physician _____

Telephone _____Fax_____

E-mail address _____

Address _____

Physician _____

Telephone _____Fax_____

E-mail address _____

Address _____

Physician _____

Telephone _____Fax_____

E-mail address _____

Address _____

To obtain copies of your hospital records:

❑ Request a copy of the medical records from the nurse manager with as much advance time as possible.

❑ Be specific about what records you are interested in obtaining, such as written reports from all or designated members of the health care team, written reports and any images of diagnostic procedures, medication sheets, surgical reports.

❑ Provide the address or fax number you want the records sent to.

❑ When necessary, be firm but polite—do not take "no" for an answer.

❑ Ask to speak with a hospital administrator or the hospital's legal counsel if you have any problems obtaining the records. Write down the names of all people you speak with.

❑ Be realistic in your timeframe expectations. The records may not be accessible as soon as you need them or expect them. Explain your reasons for any urgent need.

❑ Many hospitals will charge you a fee for copying the records. Often times, there is no fee if the records are sent to a Doctor.

❑ You can access some of your records through your doctor's or health care facility's patient portal website. Be sure to ask your doctor or health care facility for that website information.

As a patient you have the right to read your medical chart at any time. Because the chart will likely not be easy for you to understand, ask your nurse or doctor to go over it with you.

SIGNING A TREATMENT CONSENT FORM

You will have to sign a treatment consent form for a variety of invasive tests, procedures, and surgeries. Be prepared for and informed about what you are signing.

How to be prepared:

❑ Have a trusted patient advocate with you and allow the advocate to speak for you as necessary.

❑ Bring a written list of questions about the test or procedure.

❑ Bring a notebook and pen to write down any relevant information.

❑ Express any of the concerns you might have regarding the test or procedure and be sure you get the appropriate responses from the staff member.

❑ Be sure that all aspects of the test or procedure are explained to you in language you understand.

❑ Be sure to read the treatment consent form before you sign it.

❑ Signing the form with an "**X**" is legally acceptable as long as there are witnesses to verify that you were mentally competent upon signing.

❑ If you are uncomfortable with something on the form, let the staff know. Because this is a legal document, you can delete an item by crossing it out with a single line and initialing the deletion, with a brief written explanation for the deletion at the bottom of the form.

MEDICATIONS

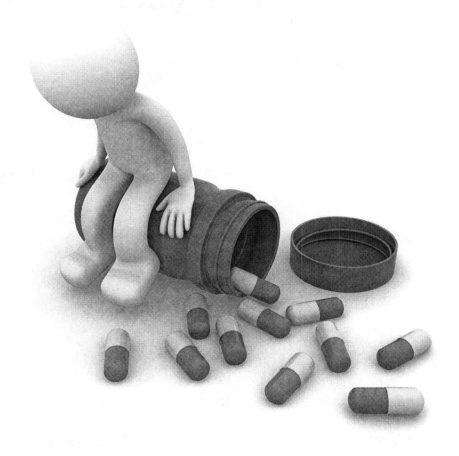

WHEN YOU'RE TAKING MEDICATION

Before take a medication know as much as possible about what it will do and why you are taking it.

Questions to ask your doctor before taking any prescription, nonprescription, herbal, over-the-counter, or supplemental medication:

❑ Why do I need the medication?

❑ What is the name of the medication?

❑ How does it work?

❑ What are the potential side effects? Which ones should I call my doctor about?

❑ Will the medication interact with other prescription and nonprescription drugs I am taking?

❑ How long will I need to be on the medication?

❑ How many times a day and at what time of the day should I take the medication?

❑ How long will it take to see the desired effects?

❑ What special information do I need to know about the drug?

☐ What allergies do I have that might cause a drug reaction?

☐ Is this drug covered on my medication prescription plan?

☐ Is this drug available in a generic form, which is usually much cheaper?

☐ What should I do if I miss a dose?

☐ Is there anything I should avoid when taking this medication?

☐ Be sure to review all medications with your primary doctor and pharmacist

☐ Be sure to read the drug informational inserts or handouts

☐ Be sure to accept all drug counseling from your local pharmacist

Remember the 3 R's for safe medication use:

1. All prescription and nonprescription medications have **risks.**

2. **Respect** the power of your medicine and the value of medicines properly used.

3. Take **responsibility** for learning about how to take your medication safely.

It is extremely important to share your health and medication history with each one of your doctors.

Bring your health history to every health care visit you have. Be sure to update it as necessary to keep it current. If you don't have your health history with you, make note of any conditions you currently have or have had, and any symptoms you are experiencing, and bring all of your medication bottles with you with the medication dosages, including herbs, supplements, and all over-the-counter drugs. **Carry a list of your medications with you at all times.**

It is critical that you use only <u>one</u> pharmacy for all of your medication needs. Pharmacists play an important role when it comes to you taking medications safely. The computer software they use will immediately alert them to any unsafe issues with the prescription or nonprescription medications that you are taking or being prescribed.

Pharmacy name _____

Address _____

Telephone number _____

MY MEDICATION CHART

DRUG	DOSE	SIDE EFFECTS	WHICH DR. PRESCRIBED IT?	WHY AM I TAKING IT?	WHAT DOES THE PILL LOOK LIKE?		

MEDICATION SAFETY AND THE ELDERLY

As people age, they become more susceptible to chronic illnesses and find themselves taking multiple drugs to treat those illnesses. With the increased use of medications comes the increased risk of drug interactions. Learn how to protect yourself!

Be sure each one of your doctors knows every prescription, nonprescription, supplemental, herbal, or over-the-counter drug you are taking, regardless of who prescribed it.

To reduce your risk of drug interactions, be sure to fill all your prescriptions at <u>one</u> pharmacy.

Pharmacy name _____

Phone number _____

Address _____

❑ Ask for medication counseling by the pharmacist.

❑ Read and **save** the written literature that comes with every prescription each time it is a filled, and refer to it if you think you are having any medication side effects.

❑ Review the written literature before you take any new medication.

❑ Call your doctor if you think you are having a side effect.

❑ Keep track of all prescription and nonprescription medications you take in the medication chart included below. Take the chart with you to **every** doctor visit.

❑ When necessary, ask someone for help in organizing your medications so they can be taken as prescribed in a safe manner.

❑ Bring your health history to every health care visit (include allergies, medications, supplements, immunizations, diseases, conditions, operations, and symptoms.) If you don't have your health history with you, make note of any conditions you currently have or have had and bring your medication chart (see below) or all of your medication bottles with you, with the medication dosages, including herbs, supplements, and over-the-counter drugs.

It is critical that you use only **one pharmacy** for all of your medication needs. Your pharmacist uses special computer software that will immediately alert him or her to any unsafe issues with the prescription or nonprescription medications you are taking.

If you miss one dose of medication, try to take the dose as soon as you remember that same day. Do not take two doses at the same time to make up for the missed dose. When in doubt, call your pharmacist or physician.

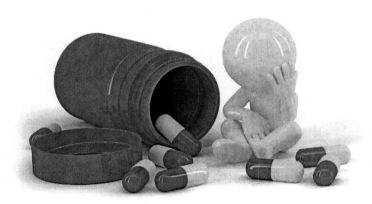

MY MEDICATION CHART

DRUG	DOSE	SIDE EFFECTS	WHICH DR. PRESCRIBED IT?	WHY AM I TAKING IT?	WHAT DOES THE PILL LOOK LIKE?

PATIENT RIGHTS AND RESPONSIBILITIES

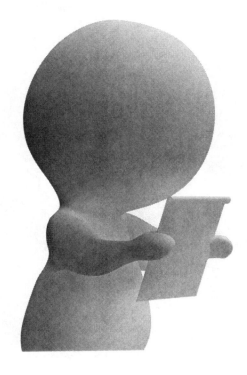

YOUR PATIENT BILL OF RIGHTS

When you assume the role of patient, regardless of your age, you have rights and responsibilities. Know what they are.

Your patient rights:

❑ Access to high quality care

❑ Respect

❑ Confidentiality to protect your privacy

❑ Personal safety

❑ Knowing the identities of health care providers

❑ Information

❑ Communication

❑ Informed consent

❑ Consultation

❑ The opportunity to refuse treatment

❑ Transfer and continuity of care

❑ Disclosure of hospital charges, and help with your billing claims

❑ Having access to hospital rules, regulations, and information

- ❏ Having grievance procedures to follow

- ❏ Participation in ethical issues

- ❏ Opportunity to have life-sustaining treatment withheld or withdrawn

- ❏ Advanced directives

- ❏ Effective pain management

- ❏ Clean, secure, and safe environments

- ❏ Involvement in your own care

- ❏ Help when you leave the hospital

- ❏ Absence of mechanical or chemical restraints

- ❏ Complete disclosure of all diagnoses, prognoses, and treatment plans

**If you feel your rights are not being met, discuss this
with your doctor, nurse, hospital patient advocacy department,
or hospital chaplain.**

Once you assume the role of patient, you also have certain responsibilities. Some of these include:

- ❏ Sharing your symptoms or changes in your symptoms with your health care team

- ❏ Complying with the recommendations of your health care team

- ❏ Taking your medication as prescribed

- ❏ Following the prescribed diet

- ❏ Following the rules of the facility

THE PATIENT CARE PARTNERSHIP

*When you become a patient, what should you expect
during your hospital stay?*

WHAT IS THE PATIENT CARE PARTNERSHIP?

The Patient Care Partnership is a document created by the American Hospital Association in 2003 that helps you as a patient understand what your expectations should be with regards to being a patient. It delineates what your patient rights are and what responsibilities you assume when you become a patient in a health care facility. There are certain things you can expect while in the hospital and there are certain things the hospital will expect from you in order for you to get better. It replaced the traditional "Patient Bill of Rights" that has been publicly posted on the walls of every health care facility for decades.

❑ If you have questions at any time, ask them. You Have a Voice... Use it.

❑ Recognize that two way communication is vital in order for you to get the best care possible.

❑ Keep a notebook and pen with you at all times. Write down your questions as they arise. Write down the answers the doctor's give you. Ask them to spell the words you can't spell. Ask them to speak in words that you can understand.

❑ Expect and demand high quality care.

❑ Expect and demand a clean and safe environment.

❑ Be involved in making decisions about your own health care.

❑ If you can't be involved, with your own care, have an Advance Directive in place that will appoint a trusted family member or friend to make medically-related decisions for you.

❑ Expect to have your privacy protected.

❑ Expect to have all discharge needs coordinated before you leave the hospital.

❑ Expect to pay your hospital bills.

For more details on The Patient Care Partnership, visit

(http://www.aha.org/aha/issues/Communicating-With-Patients/pt-care-partnership.html

Patient Responsibilities

Health care consumers are pretty savvy when it comes to their patient rights. However, they might not realize that once they assume the role of patient, along with those legally mandated rights, they also have certain responsibilities.

When you assume the role of patient, be sure you accept the responsibilities that come along with the rights:

❑ Sharing your symptoms or changes in your symptoms with your health care team

❑ Accurately sharing your past and family medical history with your health care team

❑ Complying with the recommendations of your health care team

❑ Asking for clarification of everything you do not understand

❑ Taking your medication as prescribed and questioning about the dose, the expected therapeutic effects and possible side effects

❑ Following the prescribed diet

❑ Following the prescribed activity plan

❑ Reporting any problems with your medical treatment as they arise

❑ Following the rules of the facility which include noise control, visitor control

❑ Respecting the rights and dignity of other patients

❑ Respecting the rights and dignity of your health care team

❑ Communicating with the healthcare team in a respectful and dignified manner

❑ Showing up to all therapy sessions

❑ Making sure that your bills get paid

❑ Showing up for all follow up appointments

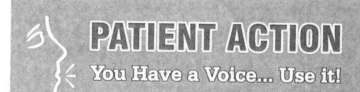

PATIENT SUPPORT

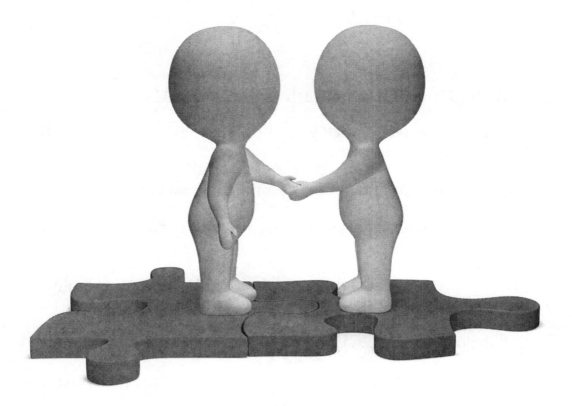

HOW TO BE A GOOD VISITOR

When you visit someone who is ill, you want to be there to help. Here are some tips to make sure that you will be the perfect visitor.

Things to consider when planning a visit:

❑ Be sure you are feeling well yourself. *Do* **not** visit if you are not feeling well.

❑ Call in advance to find out the best time for you to visit.

❑ Try to avoid visiting at meal times, unless the nurse tells you this might be helpful.

❑ Stop by the nurses' station before entering the patient's room to see if it is okay to visit.

❑ Call the patient and ask if you can bring anything for him or her.

❑ Talk to the patient's nurse about any special diet the patient might be on before you bring any food items.

❑ There is little space in the patient's room for gift items.

❑ Anything you bring to the patient needs to be transported when the patient is transferred or discharged.

- ❑ Fragrant items such as flowers, body lotion, hand cream, perfume, after-shave, and hairspray can cause nausea and vomiting in some patients.

- ❑ The visit is all about the patient and his or her needs.

What to bring on your visit:

- ❑ Handmade gift certificate for something you could do for the patient upon his or her discharge, such as delivering a meal, an IOU for a lunch date, tickets to the movies, babysitting, pet-sitting, transportation to a doctor appointment, and so on

- ❑ A game to play with the patient if she or he is up to it

- ❑ Photographs or other items to share with the patient

- ❑ Paper and pencil to write down information

- ❑ Current-event topics to talk about

- ❑ Books, magazines, puzzles, word games, or similar items

What not to bring:

- ❑ Any items that have a fragrance (creams, perfumes, hand lotions, plants, flowers, etc.)

- ❑ Allergy-aggravating items such as plants and flowers

- ❑ Anything valuable

- ❑ Food or beverages not on the patient's therapeutic diet (speak to the patient's nurse)

- ❑ Anything that will upset the patient

When you don't know what to say during your visit:

❑ Be honest. Let the patient know that you don't really know what to say or do.

❑ Let the patient know that you are there because you care.

❑ Avoid asking many questions.

❑ Ask the patient if she or he has the energy for a conversation.

❑ If the patient has no energy or is in pain, avoid lengthy conversation.

❑ Know that it is okay to just sit together in silence.

❑ Hold the patient's hand.

❑ Rub the patient's back or arm.

❑ Be present. The patient will sense that you care.

❑ Listen to what the patient says to you, and reflect back what he or she has said.

❑ Be aware of your own comfort level, but make sure that the visit is all about the patient and his or her needs.

❑ Avoid any negative conversation.

❑ It is okay to talk about topics such as the patient's hospital experience, family, job, vacations, expectations, fears, hopes, dreams,.

Know when it's time to leave:

❑ Don't stay longer than 20 minutes if the patient is not feeling well or seems sleepy.

❑ Excuse yourself from the room when a member of the patient's health care team or clergy comes in to administer care or talk with the patient.

❑ Before you depart, ask the patient if there is anything you can do for him or her.

❑ Let the nurse know when you are leaving if the patient is alone.

❑ Be sure the patient has the nurse call bell within reach.

HOW TO BE A PATIENT ADVOCATE

Being the patient's voice when the patient cannot speak is a huge responsibility. It is necessary to prepare for this role, one of the most important jobs you will ever have.

Your role as patient advocate:

❑ Let the staff know that you will be advocating for the patient.

❑ Sign any necessary patient advocacy forms.

❑ Be familiar with the patient's wishes for treatment; have copies of the patient's advance directive and DNR (do not resuscitate).

❑ Be prepared to spend time with the patient (possibly even sleeping at the patient's bedside).

❑ Find out when the health care team makes bedside rounds, and try to be there.

❑ Be prepared with written questions and concerns.

❑ Bring paper and pen for writing down important information.

❑ Be the patient's voice as needed.

❑ Ask the questions that need to be asked of all health care providers.

❑ Ask for explanations, drawings, and/or spelling of things you don't understand.

- [ ] Give explanations to the patient as needed.

- [ ] Encourage the patient to be independent.

- [ ] Encourage the patient to participate in decision making.

- [ ] Protect the patient when you feel protection is necessary.

- [ ] Find out how to best communicate with the staff when you are not at the bedside.

- [ ] Be kind and considerate of others, but be assertive in getting the patient the best care possible.

- [ ] Familiarize yourself with the facility's chain of communication in case you need to seek assistance from a higher authority.

Important questions to ask:

What is the patient's problem (diagnosis)?

If there is no diagnosis yet, how will it be made? What diagnostic tests will be ordered? Why?

What are the patient's chances of a full recovery?

Will the patient be able to return to independent living? If not, who will help the patient and family make the appropriate plans?

What medications are being given to the patient, and why? What are their dosages? What side effects should be looked for?

MY MEDICATION CHART

DRUG	DOSE	SIDE EFFECTS	WHICH DR. PRESCRIBED IT?	WHY AM I TAKING IT?	WHAT DOES THE PILL LOOK LIKE?

Items you may need:

- ❏ Sweater or jacket

- ❏ Reading materials

- ❏ Reading glasses

- ❏ Music (with earphones)

- ❏ Games/playing cards

- ❏ Snacks and drinks

- ❏ Computer and charger

- ❏ Cell phone and charger

- ❏ Notebook and writing utensil

- ❏ Comfortable clothing and shoes

- ❏ Phone numbers of patient's family and close friends

- ❏ Change of clothing and other personal items in case you are away longer than expected (including your own personal medications)

- ❏ Feel free to ask the nursing staff for a pillow, sheet and blanket and/or other necessary items if you will be spending the night.

WHY YOU NEED A PATIENT ADVOCATE

You have a voice, but if there is ever a time when you will struggle to use it, it will be in the hospital. A patient advocate will be your voice.

You might not be able to use your voice if you are in pain, under stress, anxious, frightened, under the influence of mind-altering drugs, confused, unconscious, sedated, under anesthesia, having surgery or another procedure, physically or emotionally unable to speak, or unable to speak the local language.

Every patient needs a trusted advocate. Who will yours be?

Advocate name _____

Home phone _____ Cell phone _____

Address _____

Alternate advocate name _____

Home phone _____ Cell phone _____

Address _____

The role of the patient advocate:

❑ Discuss your care with your health care team.

❑ Discuss your medications with your doctors and nurses.

❑ Be present during health care team rounds.

❑ Ask the questions you may be unable to ask.

❑ Explain and clarify what you don't understand.

❑ Discuss treatment options with your health care team.

❑ Help you understand treatment or procedure consent forms.

❑ Share your advance directive with the staff (If you do not have an advance directive, let your advocate notify the hospital that you wish to have the documents created.).

❑ Stay overnight as needed.

❑ Act as the liaison between your health care team and your family.

THE CHALLENGES OF BEING A CAREGIVER

Family caregivers face the grim reality of providing or coordinating the 24/7 care for their aging parents or other relatives. Sometimes overworked and overstressed caregivers die before the person being cared for.

How you advocate for yourself as a family caregiver:

❑ Share your situation with your employer.

❑ Share your situation with siblings, other family members, and friends, and don't refuse offers for respite/break time, meals, visits, outings, and the like. Ask for help as necessary.

❑ Solicit input and guidance from siblings, other family members, and friends who live in or out of town.

❑ Establish expectations for total family involvement in the caregiving or coordination of care.

❑ Create a financial plan and speak frankly with family members about the financial burdens of caregiving.

❑ Seek out financial counseling through personal financial advisors, bankers, local social service agencies, or Medicare/Medicaid offices.

❑ Share your situation with your clergy.

❑ Seek out community caregiving resources (church, civic, social, health care organizations; adult day-care centers, respite care, peer support; Alzheimer's Association, Alzheimer's Foundation of America, Alzheimer's Research Forum; local memory clinics/centers).

❑ Speak with your primary care provider about caregiving resources.

❑ Seek out online resources and online chats taking place on the subject of caregiving.

❑ Seek out respite from community agencies (church, social services, Alzheimer's Association).

❑ Focus on the positive aspects of caring for your loved one.

❑ Be open to outside help.

Prepare for others to care for your relative by leaving written instructions including:

❑ Brief description of medical situation

❑ Helpful care techniques

❑ Your loved one's favorite foods

❑ Feeding times

❑ Activities your loved one enjoys

❑ Any unusual behaviors of your loved one

❑ Normal disposition of your loved one

❑ Normal activities of your loved one, such as bed rest, out of bed to chair, walk to bathroom

❑ Bathroom needs

- ❏ Items that need special attention

- ❏ Family contact information

- ❏ Favorite TV shows or radio stations

- ❏ Favorite sleeping positions

- ❏ Things that stimulate your loved one in a positive way, things that upset him or her, things that please him or her, and things that calm him or her

- ❏ Keep a journal for all caregivers to document their care of your loved one

To maintain your own mental, physical, and spiritual well-being, be sure to:

- ❏ Have at least one hour each day away from the person you are caring for (respite)

- ❏ Create a schedule in advance with self-care as a priority

- ❏ Eat well-balanced meals

- ❏ Find time to exercise

- ❏ Get the sleep you require

- ❏ Allow time to do things you enjoy

- ❏ Reach out to others

- ❏ Recognize signs of stress (depression, guilt, fear, grief, sleep deprivation) in yourself and seek help as needed

- ❏ Keep a daily gratitude journal, which will allow you to focus on positive things in your life

❏ Seek out the help of local social service agencies that might be able to provide resources for care or respite for caregivers

<u>List of others who participate in caregiving:</u>

Name_____

Phone number_____

Name_____

Phone number_____

Name_____

Phone number_____

Name_____

Phone number_____

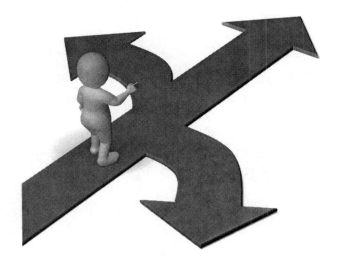

DISCHARGE PLANNING

You've been in the hospital and have had all your needs met by your health care team. It's time to go home. Now what happens?

Things you should know about discharge planning:

❏ Discharge planning is planning for the care you will need after you are discharged from a health care facility.

❏ The planning actually begins on the day you are admitted.

❏ Discharge planning involves the evaluation of and planning to meet your biological, psychological, social, and spiritual needs once you are discharged.

❏ The goal is to help you recover to your former state of health and/or help you cope with any limitations or disabilities that your illness or injury may present you with.

❏ Depending on your needs, a social worker and a home health nurse may come to your home right after your discharge to perform an initial evaluation, to determine your needs, and to plan accordingly.

❏ When necessary, the discharge planning team will provide you with a list of recommended long-term care, rehabilitation, assisted-living, or nursing home facilities.

❏ Be sure that you or your designated advocate understands the discharge instructions.

Who is involved with discharge planning?

❑ Medical social worker

❑ Discharge planning nurse specialist

❑ Home health nurse

❑ Family members or significant others

❑ Patient

Who requires discharge planning?

Patients who, after discharge, will require some assistance with activities of daily living such as bathing, food preparation, feeding, dressing, medications, walking, dressing changes, maintenance of patient-care equipment.

Who gives the post-discharge care?

❑ Home health nurses or nursing assistants or aides provided through a community home care agency

❑ Therapists (such as occupational, physical, or speech)

❑ Family or significant other as available

❑ Aides or companions hired by the patient or family

If the patient has a private home health or long-term care insurance policy, share that information with the discharge planning team so they can initiate contact with the policy provider.

EASING THE TRANSITION WHEN YOUR LOVED ONE IS PLACED IN LONG-TERM CARE

When a person leaves his or her home and independence behind for the rest of his or her life, there is a tremendous amount of loss. Learn what you can do to ease that intense emotion, both for you and your loved one.

Making the transition easier:

❑ Allow your loved one to respond with anger, depression, and/or aggression. Allow yourself to feel guilt and depression.

❑ Help your loved one say good-bye to his or her home through some type of ritual or gathering to mark the moment.

❑ Allow your loved one to supervise decisions about what to take, what to give away, and to whom things should be given.

❑ Make sure your loved one brings treasured mementos to the facility. She or he may not be able to bring furniture, but photos of loved ones and friends are welcome and comforting items to have around.

❑ Bring objects that reflect something about who your loved one has been. Bring photos of him or her taken during earlier stages of life.

❑ Mark the arrival of the "new" home with a cultural or religious ritual—for example, a mezuzah for a Jewish person, or a special crucifix for a Christian.

❑ Visit your loved one regularly, which lets him or her know that he or she has not been forgotten.

❑ Find things to do together with your loved one that she or he particularly enjoys, such as going outside to enjoy fresh air, sharing news about the family, reading poetry, or participating in a facility activity.

❑ If permitted, take your loved one out of the facility for a few hours for some recreation and diversion.

❑ Encourage your loved one to build relationships with the people in the facility and to have worthwhile experiences.

❑ Encourage your loved one to participate in the activities that are offered at the facility. Accompany them to those activities. Make it a fun time for both of you.

❑ Help your loved one find meaning in his or her daily life even though he or she may be suffering. Encourage your loved one to do something nice for someone else. Encourage him or her to say a kind word to someone else. Let your loved one know how much he or she can grow and change by interacting with others and by participating in activities.

❑ Have the grandkids call and speak with your loved one over the phone. If you have the knowledge and ability, Skype or Facetime with family members who live far away while you are visiting your loved one in the facility.

❑ Help your loved one reminisce about days gone as a tool for overcoming depression, loss, and isolation.

❑ Develop a positive relationship with the staff. Thank the staff members when appropriate and be sure to acknowledge the positive things they do to their supervisors.

❑ Get the staff to appreciate what is special about your loved one by telling them about his or her past accomplishments and strengths.

❑ Make a schedule for visits by family, friends, and members of your loved one's faith community.

❑ Be sure to inform the staff of your loved one's specific needs. Communicate, with respect and tact, any concerns you might have about your loved one's care.

❑ Report any unaddressed concerns to the facility social worker or administrator. If this doesn't bring the desired outcome, call the nursing home ombudsman, who is a federally funded advocate, through your local Area Agency on Aging. Call your State Department of Aging or look in the government section of your phone book to find the Area Agency of Aging closest to you.

❑ Take good care of yourself. Get enough sleep and eat well. Take breaks from caregiving. Consider reaching out to a support group for children of aging parents. Seek counseling from your clergy. Nurture yourself by spending quality time with family and friends, spending time by yourself, and/or pampering yourself with something that gives you pleasure and comfort.

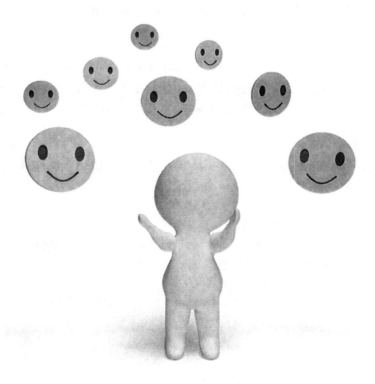

SURGICAL PROCEDURES

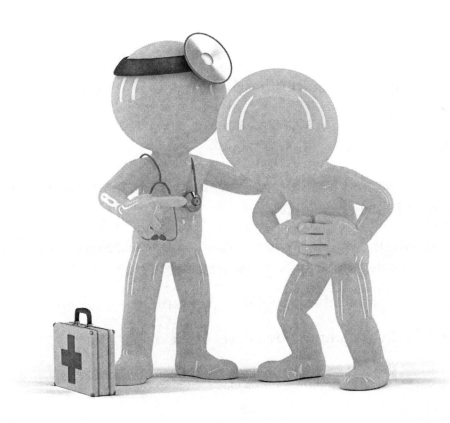

QUESTIONS TO ASK BEFORE SURGERY

The thought of having surgery is scary. Being informed is a good way to control that fear.

❏ Which surgeon is performing the procedure? Who will be assisting the surgeon?

❏ Who else will be in the operating room with me?

❏ Will all involved health care providers and laboratories be part of my health insurance network?

❏ Who will be putting me to sleep, the anesthesiologist (medical doctor) or the nurse anesthetist (registered nurse)?

❏ What type of anesthesia will be used to put me to sleep?

❏ What are the potential side effects of the anesthesia?

❏ What are the risks involved with that type of anesthesia?

❏ How long will the surgery take?

❏ How long will I be in the recovery room?

❏ What medical equipment might I expect to wake up with?

❏ How will my pain and anxiety be managed?

❏ When will my family be able to see me after my surgery?

- ❑ If a biopsy is performed, when will I find out the results? Who is responsible for sharing those results with me?

- ❑ Which member of my health care team will be the one to communicate with my family during and after surgery?

- ❑ When will I be able to get out of bed?

- ❑ When will I be able to drink fluids? Eat solid food?

- ❑ When can I expect to be discharged?

- ❑ Will I need help with me at home after discharge?

- ❑ Will I need any therapy or special equipment after surgery?

- ❑ Are there any restrictions to my activity after surgery?

- ❑ When can I return to work/school?

- ❑ When can I resume sexual activity?

- ❑ When will I need to see the surgeon again?

- ❑ When will my sutures or staples be removed? By whom?

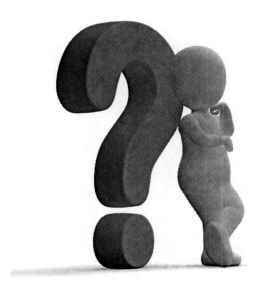

SO YOU'RE HAVING ANESTHESIA

Before you allow yourself to be put to sleep, make sure you have all the necessary facts.

Meeting with the anesthesiologist:

You will probably be scheduled to have a meeting with an anesthesiologist the week before your operation. The anesthesiologist is the medical specialist who puts you to sleep during surgery. The one you meet with is not necessarily the one who will put you to sleep during your operation.

What to bring to the meeting:

❏ A trusted patient advocate who is able to speak for you

❏ A copy of your health history (including allergies, medications, supplements, immunizations, diseases, conditions, operations, and symptoms)

❏ Your health insurance ID, Medicare, and/or Medicaid card

❏ A photo ID

❏ Paper and pen so you can write down any necessary information

❏ A written list of questions you may have about your anesthesia or surgical experience

❏ A copy of your advance directive and DNR (do not resuscitate) (See page 80)

❑ A list of any drug or food allergies

❑ Your medication containers and medication dosages, including herbs, supplements, and over-the-counter drugs, or a written list of same

Report any issues you might have with your head, neck, back, or extremities so your operating room team can consider those issues when positioning you on the operating table.

Questions to ask the anesthesiologist:

❑ Who will be in the operating room with me?

❑ Who will be putting me to sleep?

❑ What type of anesthesia will be used to put me to sleep?

❑ What are the potential side effects of the anesthesia?

❑ What are the risks involved with this type of anesthesia?

❑ How long will the surgery take?

❑ What medical equipment might I have in place upon waking up from anesthesia?

❑ How long will I be in the recovery room?

❑ How will my pain and anxiety be managed?

❑ When can my family see me after the surgery?

❑ Is the anesthesiology group in my health insurance provider network?

On the day of surgery:

❑ Bring the same items that you brought with you to the anesthesia meeting.

❑ Bring an advocate with you to be your health care proxy while you are under anesthesia.

❑ Confirm that all members of your operating team have your current medical history.

❑ Mark an **X** on the site being operated on with a permanent marker before going to the hospital to avoid any confusion on the day of surgery. Be sure the operating team sees it and confirms the site.

❑ Share any special needs you might have, or any changes in your condition or circumstances.

❑ Once again, be sure to share any issues you might have with your head, neck, back, or extremities so those issues can be considered when you are being positioned on the operating table.

❑ Question any differences between the consent form the surgeon had you sign prior to surgery and the form that the operating room staff may ask you to sign on the day of surgery.

❑ Read the consent form carefully, and question anything you don't understand. See worksheet "Signing a Treatment Consent Form." (See page 86)

SO YOU'RE HAVING SHOULDER SURGERY

Preparing for Surgery:

❏ If you are having shoulder surgery, you will probably need help with many of your activities of daily living after surgery, including bathing, toileting, dressing, and meal preparation. Make plans to have someone who is physically able to help you stay with you during your first week home, especially if you have small children who need to be picked up. It's nice to have someone there to answer your phone calls or the doorbell, if you drop something, or if something heavy has to be lifted. It's especially nice to have someone prepare your meals and to cater to you in other ways during that first week or two after your surgery.

❏ If you can't get someone to stay with you, you can prepare yourself by freezing some meals that can be easily zapped in the microwave as the need arises. Have available small containers that you can open with one hand—containers of cereal, milk, yogurt, cheese crackers, pretzels, and the sort. If you are alone, put nonperishable items and bottled water in a cooler and leave it near where you will be spending most of your time that first week. Put bottled water and other liquids that you enjoy into the refrigerator. Have your significant other or child prepare your lunch and beverages and put them in a cooler so you have easy access.

❏ Buy paper plates, cups, and plastic eating utensils to use when you are alone.

❏ Make sure you have a phone nearby (cell or cordless phone), or hook your phone up to an answering machine so you don't have to answer every call. You can retrieve messages when you are up to it. Don't feel obligated to call people back during the first week after surgery. People just want to let you know that they are thinking of you, and most will understand that you aren't up to talking on the phone or retrieving messages.

❑ Buy one of those long grasper tools that you can pick things up with without having to bend down. They cost about $7 and can be purchased at most retail drug stores. They're also good for retrieving items off of high shelves or cabinets, but you shouldn't be doing this after you've had shoulder surgery!

❑ If you have health insurance, call the insurance company and find out if you are entitled to any home health care. If you have long-term care insurance, you may also be entitled to home health care, depending on your policy and the extent of your surgery.

❑ Buy yourself a lap, or a clipboard for reading. You can turn the pages using one hand. Make a pile of the magazines and books you haven't had the time to read. You probably won't have the energy or desire to read during your first week or two home, but after that, reading helps to pass the time.

❑ Have a radio and/or TV (with remote) near where you will be spending much of your recuperation. It helps pass the time.

❑ Have a notebook so you can write down the names of those who send you gifts, flowers, meals, and the like, or who visit you, so you can send them thank-you notes later on. You may also use this notebook for journaling your thoughts as you get stronger. It is very useful to write down things that you are grateful for each day—it takes the emphasis away from feeling sorry for yourself.

❑ Let everyone important to you know about your operation in advance. Tell them the exact date and time of the operation, and ask them to send you loving and positive thoughts and prayers at the very moment your operation starts.

❑ If anyone asks you how they can help, ask them to bring over a dinner that you can put in your freezer. Ask them to drive you to physical therapy, the doctor, or the store, or to run errands for you. Ask them to visit when you are ready for that.

- ❑ Learn to ask others for help. When people ask what they can do for you, let them know exactly what you need. Make a list of the names and phone numbers of people who offer to help, and keep it handy.

- ❑ Buy some lavender oil. Research shows that the fragrance of lavender sends a calming message to the brain, which counters adrenaline-producing stress signals. Lavender can be purchased in many health-food stores.

- ❑ By the time you opt for surgery, you will have probably acquired a variety of pillows to help you sleep. These will be put to good use after your surgery.

- ❑ Purchase items such as soap, shampoo, and conditioner with pumps. These will be easier to use with one hand.

- ❑ Buy a handheld showerhead. This will allow you to shower without getting your sutures wet and will make showering easier for you once your sutures are removed. Don't go for the cheapest one—they leak. Set it up before your surgery so you will know that it fits in your shower and doesn't leak.

- ❑ If needed, obtain a sturdy shower chair for the shower. A cheap plastic chair will work, but make sure it is sturdy. You don't want to have an accident in the shower.

- ❑ Put all of the personal items you use daily in an open container so you will have easy access.

- ❑ Buy toothpaste that has a flip top that can be easily manipulated with one hand.

- ❑ If you like to use dusting powder, buy powder in a container with a mitt that can be manipulated with one hand.

- ❑ Buy **flushable** personal wipes and put a container in each bathroom. They will help you feel clean, especially during the period when you cannot shower. Be sure they are flushable, or they will clog up your toilet.

❑ Buy facial wipes for cleaning your face. They are far easier to use with one hand than trying to wash your face using soap and water. Check to see if they are flushable.

❑ Hang a large bath sheet on a hook in your bathroom. You can back up against it to dry your own back.

❑ Buy a box of powdered laundry detergent and cut the lid off. Use a small plastic cup for scooping up the detergent when you feel up to doing laundry. This will make it easier to manipulate with one hand.

❑ Make a pile of clothing that you will be wearing for the next month or so, including elastic-banded loose-fitting pants/shorts, extra-large tee shirts that will fit over your splint, socks that are easy to put on, slip-on shoes/sneakers, underwear, and the like. It's a lot easier than having to go into your closet or dresser each day. Ladies, don't worry about wearing bras for quite some time. If you absolutely cannot go without a bra, go on the internet and research strapless bras. You should also research silicon bra cups. This is a new type of bra that is strapless and backless and very comfortable. They retail for about $20 each. Be sure the tee shirts you get are large enough to slip over your surgical splint, as you won't be able to put your arm through the arm hole.

❑ Prepare a pile of blank thank-you cards so you can start writing them when you have the energy. Be sure to have stamps in the house.

❑ You will be icing your shoulder after surgery. Speak to your doctor about this. She or he can give you a prescription for a continuous icing machine which you can purchase at any medical supply store. Medical supply stores also sell ice packs for such purposes, but they can be costly. The most effective icing is done with the icing machine, but you can save money by making your own ice packs. Make three ice packs before your surgery so you will always have one available:

Fill a gallon-size ziplock plastic bag with water and rubbing alcohol, in a 2:1 ratio (2 parts of water for every part of alcohol—2 cups of water to one cup of alcohol). Put them in the freezer.

OR

Fill a gallon-size ziplock bag with green Palmolive dish detergent, leaving 2 inches of space for expansion during freezing.

Be sure to protect your skin with a cloth barrier before placing an ice pack against it.

❑ You may also be applying heat to your shoulder prior to doing physical therapy. You can make a heat pack by filling up a high sock about two-thirds of the way with any kind of rice and tying it in a knot. Then "cook" the sock in the microwave for 45 -60 seconds. It will be hot! Be careful not to burn yourself. If the sock is long enough, you will be able to wrap the sock around your shoulder joint.

❑ If you will be going to an outpatient physical therapy center, you will need to make arrangements for people to transport you, as you will not be able to drive for a few weeks. If you have no one to drive you, let your therapy center and doctor know. You might find some volunteers at your synagogue or church who can help. If you have a neighbor with small children, trade transportation for babysitting services once you are feeling better. If your neighbor couldn't use babysitting services, figure out what you can offer in return for the neighbor taking you to therapy. If you don't have transportation, check with your health insurance company to see if you are eligible for physical therapy at home.

❑ If you have no one to shop for you after surgery, fill up your pantry, freezer, and refrigerator with desired and necessary items before your surgery.

❑ If you normally take medications each day, make sure you have enough to get you through your recuperation period (probably about 6–8 weeks). Buy a pill box that will allow you to prepare your meds in advance for 2 weeks so they will be easily accessible to you. You can also pour each of your medications into a separate small ziplock plastic bag for easy access. Be sure to put the medication container in the plastic bag so you will know which drug is which. You should also label the bag with the drug name, dose, and time(s) it should be taken. Be very careful about doing this if there are small children in the home.

❑ If you are going to be hospitalized and you have a favorite pillow that you usually sleep on, you may want to bring it with you for comfort. Be sure to bring a brightly colored pillowcase(s) with you so the staff will know that the pillow is yours and so it won't end up on another patient's bed!

❑ Prepare advance directives and bring them with you. If you don't have these documents, go to **www.putitinwriting.org** and obtain them or let your nurse know you want to fill these documents out. (see page 80)

❑ Ask someone you trust to be your patient advocate and to accompany you for surgery so he or she can speak for you when you can't use your own voice. The surgery will be not be performed if you do not have an advocate. For a same day surgical procedure, your advocate will also need to drive you home, as you won't be able to drive yourself.

❑ Discuss the use of magnet therapy with your doctor. Magnets increase blood circulation and can promote healing. Small "spot" magnets are perfect for surgical incisions as they can be placed around your incision as soon as the bulky bandages are removed. They can be held in place with small round Band-Aids and can be worn for one to two weeks post-op. They can get wet and can be reapplied with more Band-Aids. They can be purchased online at websites such as **www.promagnet.com**.

On surgery day:

❑ Wear pants with an elastic waistband to the hospital or surgery center, and slip-on shoes. These will make it easier to get dressed after the surgery when you can only use one arm. Be sure to bring an extra-large (or extra-extra-large) tee shirt with you to wear home that will slip over your surgical splint. Bring your personal items and clean underwear with you if there's a chance you might be spending the night in the hospital.

❑ You will be admitted to a pre-op area, where you will be assigned a nurse who will admit you. An intravenous (IV) line will be started for the administration of fluids and drugs during your surgery. You will be seen by the anesthesiologist. Report any head, neck, back, or related problems so extra attention can be paid to the positioning of your body during the operation. You will also be visited by your surgeon. This is the time to ask any last-minute questions.

❑ You will most likely be asked to sign an informed consent for the surgery unless you have already signed one. When you sign this form, it indicates that you understand the procedure being performed and the possible risks. Be sure to ask for clarification if you don't understand what you are agreeing to.

❑ If you feel really nervous, put some lavender oil on your forearm and take a big whiff of its fragrance. Do some deep breathing, breathing in through your nose and out through your mouth.

❑ If you are so inclined, ask your doctor, nurse, and family to say a prayer with you for a good outcome. Visit **www.PatientAction.com** and click on the **PRAYER** link to access many appropriate prayers for such purpose.

❑ Tell your loved one or other patient advocate who accompanies you to surgery to bring a jacket, reading materials, cell phone with charger, laptop with charger, music, and something to eat or drink with them.

During the first few days after surgery:

❑ Continue to use your lavender as needed. Stroke a drop of it over your temples to reduce tension headaches; massage a drop across the exterior of your throat to calm tickly coughs; place a drop on the pillow to relieve insomnia. Put some on your forearm so you can keep smelling it to reduce stress.

❑ If you planned on using magnets, ask someone to place your magnets around your incision as soon as possible after your bulky bandages are removed. If the magnets fall off, reapply them with new circular Band-Aids. You can get them wet.

❑ Your throat may be sore after surgery. This soreness is due to the breathing tube they insert into your throat during surgery while you were asleep. Your doctor can order a throat spray if the soreness is very uncomfortable. Throat lozenges or lollipops can also help.

❏ You do have a voice! Be your own advocate! Don't be afraid to ask questions. Write them down so you won't forget to ask them when you see your doctor. If you have a patient advocate with you, have your advocate write down your questions and have him or her ask the questions for you if you are unable to ask them yourself.

❏ Be aware of the major role that hand washing plays in the control of infection. Wash your hands frequently, and make sure your health care team washes their hands before touching you! Don't be afraid to remind them to do this. Hand washing between patients is an industry standard.

❏ Don't be afraid to cough, even if it hurts. Coughing reduces your risk of pulmonary complications, such as pneumonia.

❏ Most shoulder surgery is performed arthroscopically, which involves tiny quarter-inch incisions for the passage of instruments into your shoulder joint. There is no major incision and no suturing with arthroscopic surgery. If your surgery is not going to be arthroscopic, you will probably have a larger incision with surgical sutures that will need to be removed. Do not worry about their removal. It really doesn't hurt! If you feel very anxious, do some deep breathing, breathing in through your nose and out through your mouth during the removal. Plan your pain medication to coincide with the timing of the removal. Take a whiff of lavender to relax you.

❏ See if your doctor is willing to give you your prescriptions for post-op medications a day or two before surgery or hospital discharge so you can have them in the house upon your arrival home from the hospital. Keep your medications nearby once you go home so they are easily accessible to you. If you don't have to worry about small children getting into your medications, ask the pharmacist for container tops that are easily opened. You can also dump your pills into a small ziplock plastic bag for easy one-handed accessibility. Make sure you leave the pill container in the bag so you can identify the pills. Label the bags in advance with medication name, dose, and time(s) to be taken.

❑ Narcotic pain medication prescriptions cannot be refilled or re-ordered over the phone. You will need to have someone go to your doctor's office to pick up a new prescription. Be sure to have enough pain medication on hand to cover your pain needs for any weekends or holidays when your doctor's office may be closed.

❑ Discuss post-op bowel function with your doctor, *especially* if you tend to be constipated. The anesthesia, decreased activity, and pain medication will predispose you to constipation. It can be a real problem. Make sure you have what you need at home before your surgery. Find out what you can use, and use it!

❑ If you are hospitalized, plan to take your last dose of pain medication about 45 minutes **before** you leave the hospital for home. It will help ease the discomfort during the ride home.

Once you are home:

❑ Carefully follow all of your doctor's instructions!

❑ You may continue to have what the doctors call referred pain in your upper arm on the operated side for many weeks post-op. Don't be afraid to speak with your doctor about pain management. Don't be a martyr. You don't need to suffer. Icing helps a lot. Take your pain medications as prescribed for at least the first two weeks. It's important to stay on top of the pain. You may even want to set your alarm so you can keep on top of the pain during the night. This will help you recover more quickly, as your body can focus on healing, not on coping with pain. Keep your pain medications and water close by so you can easily reach them. (Be careful to make sure that young children do not have access to them.) Do not drive or operate any dangerous equipment or machinery while taking pain medications.

❑ Adequate rest is important for your recovery, but sleeping can be a real problem for you both pre- and post-operatively as you toss and turn, trying to find a comfortable place for your affected arm. It is not uncommon for patients to have problems sleeping after they go off their pain medications. Let your doctor know if you are having trouble sleeping.

Your doctor may consider prescribing something to help you sleep. Sleeping in a recliner both pre- and post-op may be the best thing you can do for yourself. If you don't have one, you can rent one by the week or month from your local medical supply store. Do the research before your surgery so if you need one, it is only a phone call away. Ask if the chair comes with an electric seat elevator. That can be really helpful. If a recliner is not an option for you, prop yourself up with several pillows.

❑ If you sleep on your back, try positioning a pillow under your affected arm. A pillow under your knees may also help you get more comfortable. A body pillow can also be helpful. They can be purchased at many retail stores (Walmart, Target, and Bed, Bath & Beyond, for example) Buy a pillowcase to fit the body pillow so you can launder it as needed.

❑ If possible (or desirable), sleep alone the first week so you have the full space in your bed to get yourself comfortable.

❑ Make a list of any questions you might want to ask your doctor at your first post-op visit, which usually takes place within 7–10 days after surgery. Your sutures will probably be removed at this visit.

❑ Time your pain medication so you take it about 45 minutes prior to any outings.

❑ If you feel you must shower before you are allowed to get your incisions wet, cut an inexpensive slicker in half so it will cover your shoulder area. You'll have to hold it tightly around your neck to prevent the water from getting in, but it will be worth the effort to be able to shower. You'll be able to shampoo using the slicker, too. Don't forget to use a plastic chair in the shower if necessary. The use of a handheld showerhead will come in handy here, especially if someone is helping you with your shower.

❑ **Physical therapy is critical to your complete recovery!** It is no picnic, but you must actively participate. The pain you experience during therapy is normal. Take your pain medication about 45 minutes prior to therapy, which will reduce your pain and help maximize your therapy session. Don't expect an overnight recovery. It takes a good 6 weeks of therapy to see any real progress. Be patient. Be persistent. Be committed to your therapy. Keep icing!

Call your doctor immediately if you have any of the following symptoms:

- ❏ Fever

- ❏ Sweats

- ❏ Redness around or drainage from your incision

- ❏ Shaking chills

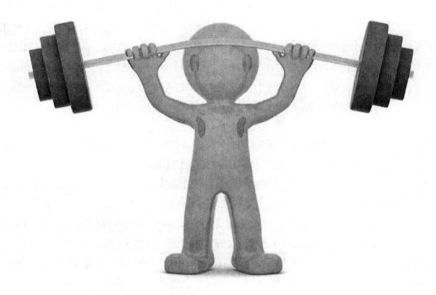

SO YOU'RE HAVING ABDOMINAL SURGERY

Preparing for your surgery:

❏ Make plans to have someone stay with you during your first week home, especially if you have small children who need to be picked up. It's nice to have someone there to answer your phone calls or the doorbell, if you drop something, or if something heavy has to be lifted. It's especially nice to have someone prepare your meals and to cater to you in other ways during that first week or two.

❏ If you normally take medications each day, make sure you have enough to get you through your recuperation period. Buy a pill box that will allow you to prepare your medicines in advance for a 2-week period so they will be easily accessible to you. If you are weak from the surgery and having a difficult time opening the tops of your medication containers, dump each container into its own small ziplock baggie so you can access it easily. Be sure to place the empty medicine container in the plastic bag so you can identify the medicine and know what the proper dose will be.

❏ Make sure you have a phone nearby, or hook your phone up to an answering machine so you can retrieve messages when you aren't up to answering the phone. Don't think you have to answer the phone each time it rings. You are recuperating from a major body trauma. Take the time necessary to heal.

❏ Make a pile of the magazines and books you haven't had the time to read. You probably won't have the energy or desire to read during your first week home, but after that, reading helps to pass the time. You may want to buy a lap desk to help support the book or magazine you are reading. A simple clipboard will work also.

❑ Have a radio and/ or TV (with remote!) near where you will be spending much of your recuperation. You will have much downtime during the first two weeks post-op. The distraction of radio or TV will help you pass the time.

❑ Have a notebook so you can write down the names of those who send you gifts, flowers, and the like, or who visit you, so you can send them thank-you notes. You may also use this notebook for journaling your thoughts as you get stronger. It is very therapeutic to write down things that you are grateful for each day; it takes the emphasis away from feeling sorry for yourself to being grateful each day.

❑ Plan your wardrobe for the first few weeks post-op. Loose-fitting and/or elastic-waist clothing is best. It may be difficult to wear pants for a few weeks after surgery. Make a pile of comfortable clothes so you don't have to go in and out of your closet and dresser each day.

❑ Discuss the use of magnet therapy with your doctor. Magnets increase blood circulation and can promote healing. Small "spot" magnets are perfect for surgical incisions as they can be placed around your incision as soon as the bulky bandages are removed. They can be held in place with small round Band-Aids and can be worn for one to two weeks post-op. They can get wet and can be reapplied with more Band-Aids. They can be purchased online at websites such as **www.promagnet.com**.

❑ Let everyone important to you know about your procedure in advance. Tell them the exact date and time of the operation, and ask them to send you loving and positive thoughts and prayers at the very moment you will be having your procedure. This includes your clergy.

❑ If anyone asks you how they can help, don't be shy. Tell them what you will need them to do—perhaps bring over a dinner that you can put in your freezer for when you come home, or perhaps run errands for you post-op. Write down the names and phone numbers of the people who offer to help so you can call them when you need their help.

❑ Buy some lavender oil to use while in the hospital. Research shows that the fragrance of lavender sends a calming message to the brain, which counters adrenaline-producing stress signals.

❑ Buy a full-sized body pillow (and pillowcase) that you can use at home to get yourself into a comfortable position while in bed. They can be purchased at a variety of retails shops, including Walmart. You may also want to buy a smaller foam half-round pillow, which can be invaluable for comfort while in the hospital. Purchase pillows with removable covers for washing, or use pillowcases.

❑ Bring your own pillow with brightly colored pillowcase to the hospital, as hospital pillows can be very uncomfortable. The brightly covered pillowcase will alert your health care team that this is your personal pillow while brightening up your bedside environment. Use the pillow as a splint across your incision on the car ride home to protect it from bumps along the way.

❑ Bring your favorite music to the hospital. Music is very soothing and relaxing. It can distract you from stress and discomfort. Be sure to label it with your name.

❑ While you are asleep during surgery, the anesthesiologist will be inserting a breathing tube down your throat. (Don't worry, it will be removed before you wake up!) Bring some lollipops and/or throat lozenges to the hospital with you. Once you are allowed to eat, they can be used to soothe your throat if it is sore from the tube. If the pain is moderate to severe, ask your doctor for something to help.

❑ Wear loose-fitting clothing to the hospital and then plan on wearing these same items home. You will not need a nightgown, pajamas, or bathrobe. Hospital gowns are easiest, and a second one can be used as a robe. Bring comfortable slip-on rubber-soled slippers or sandals. Try not to walk barefoot in the hospital. Bring a pair of flip-flops for the shower.

❑ Bring a toothbrush and toothpaste. Mouthwash is sometimes available from the hospital, but not always. Chapstick is extremely helpful for the first day or two, when your lips will feel really dry.

- Bring paper and pencil so you can write down all of your questions as they arise. This ensures that all of your questions can be asked and answered.

- If your doctor approved of your use of magnets, bring them with you to the hospital. Tell your advocate to place them around your incision(s) as soon as possible after your surgery.

On the day of surgery:

- Plan on having a trusted advocate accompany you to the hospital and stay with you during the surgery. The surgery will not be performed if you don't have an advocate with you. In addition, you shouldn't drive yourself to the hospital, as you will probably be stressed out. Second, as a patient, you absorb a lot less information when you are anxious, vulnerable, in pain, afraid, and/or undressed. Plan on keeping your patient advocate with you at all times, even overnight if you are going to need hospitalization. You will rest much better. Your advocate can ask questions that you may not think about when you are stressed or in pain. She or he will help you get the right medicines and treatments. Your advocate can also help remember answers to questions you have already asked. She or he can speak for you when you cannot speak for yourself. Make sure this person knows the kind of care you want. Make sure she or he knows what you want done about life support and other life-saving efforts in the event that you are unconscious and not likely to get better. Go over the consents for treatment with your advocate. Make sure you both understand exactly what you are about to agree to. Make sure your advocate knows the type of care you will need when you get home. Your advocate should know what to look for if your condition is getting worse. She or he should also know which family and friends are available to call on for help.

- Take your advance directive with you. If you don't have these documents prepared, go to **www.putitinwriting.org** and create them for yourself. These documents will speak for you when you are unable to speak for yourself. If you don't have an advance directive prepared, you can also speak with the hospital staff for help upon arriving at the hospital. (see page 80)

❑ You will be admitted to a pre-op area, where you will be assigned a nurse who will admit you. An intravenous line (IV) will be started through which you will received fluids and drugs during your surgery. You will be seen by the anesthesiologist. She or he will talk with you and explain what type of anesthesia will be used to put you to sleep. Be sure to share if you have any neck or back problems so extra attention will be paid to the positioning of your head during the operation.

❑ You may be in the pre-op area for a long time before being taken to the operating room (OR). You will probably have your IV inserted long before your surgery begins. You can get up and go to the bathroom with the IV. Ask your nurse to show you how to do that the first time. Don't be afraid to ask. Don't be afraid to go to the bathroom! Be sure to also ask the nurse for a second hospital gown that you can throw over your shoulders to maintain modesty and prevent exposure of your rear parts.

❑ If you feel really nervous, put some lavender oil on your forearm and take a big whiff of its fragrance. Do some deep breathing, breathing in through your nose and out through your mouth. If there's time, listen to some of your relaxing music.

❑ If you are so inclined, ask your doctor, nurse, and/or family to say a prayer with you for a good outcome. Visit **www.PatientAction.com** and click on the **PRAYER** link for some appropriate prayers for such purpose.

After surgery:

❑ Continue to use your lavender as needed. Stroke a drop of it over your temples to reduce tension headaches; massage a drop across your throat to calm tickly coughs; place a drop on the pillow to relieve insomnia. Put some on your forearm so you can keep smelling it to reduce stress.

❏ If your doctor approved of the use of magnets, ask your advocate or nurse to place your magnets around your incision as soon as possible after your operation. They can be applied with Band-Aids. If the magnets fall off, reapply them with new Band-Aids. It's OK to get them wet.

❏ Let your nurse know if your throat is very sore after surgery. The doctor can order a throat spray for the discomfort. Once again, this soreness is due to the breathing tube that was inserted in your throat while you were asleep during surgery.

❏ Don't be afraid to ask questions. Write them down if necessary so you won't forget to ask them when your doctor makes rounds.

❏ Be aware of the role that hand washing plays in controlling infection. Wash your hands frequently, and make sure your health care team washes their hands before touching you! Don't be afraid to remind them to do this.

❏ Get up and walk. It may hurt, but it will reduce your risk for post-op complications. If you feel weak, ask for assistance.

❏ Keep a pillow nearby at all times to hold against (splint) your incision in case you have to cough or sneeze. Don't be afraid to cough; coughing is good post-op—it reduces your risk of lung complications.

❏ Use the handheld breathing device at your bedside every hour while you're awake. This too is very important in the prevention of post-op lung complications.

❏ Ask the nurses to help position you comfortably. This may require 4–5 pillows! When you turn on your side, place a pillow against your abdomen for support, and also put one between your knees to reduce the tension on your abdomen. Turn and position yourself from side to side frequently if possible. If you need help doing this, call the nurse to help you.

❏ While you are asleep during surgery, a tube will be passed through your urethra into your bladder to drain urine during the operation.

The tube will usually be removed before you wake up. On rare occasions, having had this tube in place may interfere with the normal ability to urinate for a few hours after its removal. **It is very important for you to tell your nurse the first time you urinate (pee) after your surgery.**

❑ Do not stress out when your doctor tells you that the staples that are holding your wound together are going to be removed. It shouldn't hurt, but if you feel anxious, you can time your pain medication about 45 minutes before the staples are to be removed. You can also do some deep breathing, breathing in through your nose and out through your mouth, or take a whiff of lavender to help you relax during the removal of the staples.

❑ Ask your doctor if she or he would be willing to give you your prescriptions for post-op medications a day or two before you are discharged so someone can have them filled and ready for you upon discharge.

❑ Don't go home without discussing post-op bowel function with your doctor, especially if you tend to be constipated. Find out what you can use, and use it!

❑ Ask your doctor if there is anything you can put on your scar to promote healing and reduce scarring, but **put nothing on your incision without your doctor's approval**—especially if your incision is red, very painful, or oozing.

For the trip home:

❑ Plan to take your last dose of pain medication about 45–60 minutes before you leave the hospital for home. It will help ease the discomfort during the ride home.

❑ Hold your pillow tightly against your abdomen on the way home from the hospital. It will help protect you from the seatbelt and from any bumpiness on the way home.

Once you are home:

❑ Follow all of your doctor's instructions.

❑ Get plenty of rest.

❑ Keep all post-op doctor appointments.

❑ Don't be a martyr. You don't need to suffer. Take your pain medications as prescribed for at least the first 2 weeks. It's important to stay on top of the pain. You may even want to set your alarm so you can keep on top of the pain during the night. This will help you recover more quickly, as your body can focus on healing, not on coping with pain. Keep your pain medications and water close by so you can easily reach them. (Be careful to make sure that young children do not have access to them.) Do not drive or operate any dangerous equipment or machinery while taking pain medications.

❑ Narcotic pain medication prescriptions cannot be refilled or re-ordered over the phone. You will need to have someone go to your doctor's office to pick up a new prescription. Be sure to have enough pain medication in hand to cover your pain needs for any weekends or holidays when your doctor's office may be closed.

❑ Let your doctor know if you are having trouble sleeping. Adequate rest is important for you. Once you go off your pain medication, you may have trouble falling asleep or staying asleep. Let your doctor know. She or he may consider prescribing you something for a few days to help you sleep.

❑ Let your doctor know if you are constipated.

❑ If you sleep on your back, try positioning pillows under your thighs and/or knees, which will take some of the pressure off of your incision. Sleeping flat may be uncomfortable. Use several pillows to increase your comfort. If possible and desirable, sleep alone the first week so you have the full space in your bed to get yourself comfortable.

Call your doctor immediately if you have any of the following symptoms:

❏ Fever

❏ Sweats

❏ Redness around or drainage from your incision

❏ Abdominal pain

❏ Shaking chills

❏ Cloudy, bad-smelling urine

❏ Painful urination

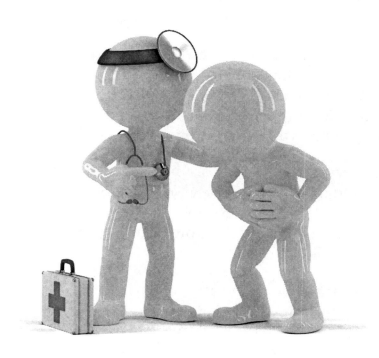

SO YOU'RE HAVING KNEE SURGERY

Preparing for surgery:

❑ Make plans to have someone who is physically able to help you stay with you during your first few days. It's nice to have someone there to answer your phone calls or the doorbell, if you drop something, or if something heavy has to be lifted. It's especially nice to have someone prepare your meals and cater to you in other ways during those first few days.

❑ If you can't get someone to stay with you, you can prepare yourself by freezing some meals that can be easily zapped in the microwave as the need arises. Have small, light containers available that you can open easily filled with cereal, milk, yogurt, cheese crackers, pretzels, and the like. If you are alone, put nonperishable items and bottled water in a container or cooler near where you will be spending most of your time that first week you are home. Put bottled water or small containers of other liquids you enjoy in the refrigerator. Have your spouse or a friend or family member prepare your lunch and beverages and put them in a cooler so you have easy access.

❑ Have paper plates, cups, and plastic eating utensils accessible for when you are alone.

❑ Make sure you have a phone nearby, or hook your phone up to an answering machine so you can retrieve messages when you are up to it.

❑ If you have medical insurance, call the insurance company and find out if you are entitled to any home health care. If you have long-term care insurance, you may also be entitled to home health care, depending on your policy and the extent of your surgery.

❏ Buy yourself a lap board with a clip on it to hold papers, books, or magazines in place. Make a pile of the magazines and books you haven't had the time to read. You probably won't have the energy or desire to read during your first few days at home, but after that, reading helps to pass the time.

❏ Have a radio and/or TV (with remote!) near where you will be spending much of your recuperation. It helps pass the time.

❏ Have a notebook handy so you can write down the names of those who send you gifts, flowers, meals, and the like, or visited you, so you can send them thank-you notes later. You may also use this notebook for journaling your thoughts as you get stronger. Some people find it very useful to write down things that they are grateful for each day; it shifts the emphasis away from feeling sorry for yourself to being grateful each day.

❏ Let everyone important to you know about your procedure in advance. Tell them the exact date and time of the operation, and ask them to send you loving and positive thoughts and prayers at the very moment you will be having your procedure. This includes your clergy.

❏ If anyone asks you how to help, ask the person to bring over a dinner that you can put in your freezer for when you come home, or ask if he or she will be able to drive you to physical therapy, the doctor, or the store or to run errands for you.

❏ Learn to ask others for help. When people ask what they can do for you, let them know exactly what you need. Make a list of the names and phone numbers of people who offer to help, and keep it handy.

❏ Buy some lavender oil. Research shows that the fragrance of lavender sends a calming message to the brain, which counters adrenaline-producing stress signals. Lavender can be purchased in many retail stores.

❏ By the time you opt for surgery, you will likely have acquired a variety of pillows to help you sleep. These will be put to good use post-operatively.

❑ Buy a handheld showerhead. This will allow you (or your caregiver) to wash yourself without getting your sutures wet and will make showering easier for you once your sutures are removed. Don't buy the cheapest one—they leak. Set up the showerhead before your surgery so you will know that it fits in your shower and that it doesn't leak.

❑ Obtain a sturdy shower chair for the shower. A cheap plastic chair will work, but make sure it is sturdy. You don't want to have an accident in the shower.

❑ Put all the personal items you use daily in an open container so you will have easy access.

❑ Buy **flushable** personal wipes and put a container in each bathroom you use. These will help you feel clean, especially during the period when you cannot shower.

❑ Hang a large bath sheet on a hook in your bathroom. You can back up against it in order to dry your own back.

❑ If you normally use liquid laundry detergent, buy a box of powdered detergent and cut the lid off. It will be easier to manipulate.

❑ Prepare a pile of thank-you cards and stamps so you can start writing the notes when you have the energy.

❑ Discuss the use of magnet therapy with your doctor. Magnets increase blood circulation and can promote healing. You can buy small "spot" magnets, which you can place around your incision as soon as the bulky bandages are removed. They can be used over and over again and can be held in place with small round Band-Aids. You can wear them for a few weeks post-op. They can get wet. They can be purchased on line at websites such as **www.promagnet.com**.

❑ You will be icing your knee post-operatively. Medical supply stores sell some really great icing products, such as a continuous ice machine for such purposes. Ice machines can be costly but they are the most effective device to use for icing. You can also use bags of frozen peas (keep refreezing them as they thaw) or make your own ice packs and save money. Make at least three ice packs so you always have one available:

Fill a gallon-size ziplock plastic bag with water and rubbing alcohol, in a 2:1 ratio (2 parts of water for every part of alcohol—2 cups of water to one cup of alcohol, for example). Freeze.

Another option is to fill a gallon-size ziplock bag with liquid green Palmolive dish washing detergent, leaving about 2 inches of dead space for expansion. Freeze.

Be sure to place a cloth barrier between your ice pack and skin to prevent skin damage.

You may also probably be applying heat to your knee prior to doing physical therapy. You can make a heat pack by filling up a high sock about 2/3 of the way with rice and tying it in a knot and then cooking it in the microwave for about 45-60 minutes. Be careful not to burn yourself it is too hot. If the sock is long enough, you will be able to wrap it around your knee joint.

❑ If you will be going to an outpatient physical therapy center, you will need to make arrangements for people to transport you if you will be unable to drive for any length of time. If you have no one to drive you, let your doctor know. You can also call your faith community or the center where you will be having physical therapy for help; they often have volunteers for such purpose. Trade transportation with a neighbor for babysitting or other such services once you've recuperated. If you are unable to find transportation, call your health insurance company and see if you are eligible for in home physical therapy.

❑ If you have no one to shop for you after surgery, fill up your pantry, freezer, and refrigerator with desired and necessary items before your surgery.

❑ If you normally take medications each day, make sure you have enough to get you through your recuperation period. Buy a pill box that will allow you to prepare your medications in advance for a 2-week period so they will be easily accessible to you.

On surgery day:

❏ Bring a tooth brush, toothpaste, a hairbrush, and a clean pair of underwear if you might be spending the night in the hospital. Plan on wearing home the same clothes you wore to the hospital. A skirt or pants with an elastic waist may be best.

❏ You will be admitted to a pre-op area, where you will be assigned a nurse who will admit you. An intravenous line (IV) will be started through which you will receive fluids and drugs. You will be seen by the anesthesiologist. Be sure to share if you have any neck problems so extra attention will be paid to the positioning of your head during the operation.

❏ If you feel really nervous, put some lavender oil on your forearm and take a big whiff of its fragrance. Do some deep breathing, breathing in through your nose and out through your mouth.

❏ If you are so inclined, ask your doctor, nurse, and/or family to say a prayer with you. Visit **www.PatientAction.com** and click on the **PRAYER** link to access many appropriate prayers for such purpose.

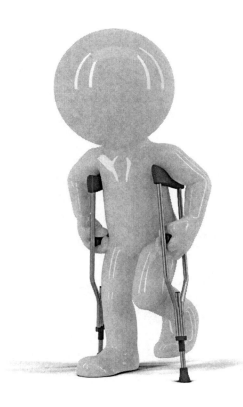

❏ Tell your loved one or other patient advocate who accompanies you to surgery to bring reading material and something to eat or drink.

❏ Bring your advance directive with you (If you do not have one prepared, go to **www.putitinwriting.org** and create one for yourself.), or tell your doctor or nurse that you want to obtain one. (see page 80)

After surgery:

❑ Continue to use your lavender as needed. Stroke a drop of it over your temples to reduce tension headaches; massage a drop across your throat to calm tickly coughs; place a drop on your pillow to relieve insomnia. Put some on your forearm so you can keep smelling it to reduce stress.

❑ If your doctor approved the use of magnets, ask your advocate or nurse to place them around your incision as soon as possible after your bulky bandages are removed. You can get the magnets wet. You can reapply with small bandaids.

❑ Don't be afraid to ask questions. Write them down so you won't forget to ask them when you see your doctor. Ask your doctor to speak in language you can understand if that is an issue for you.

❑ Be aware of the role of hand washing in controlling infection. Wash your hands frequently, and make sure your health care team and your visitors wash their hands before touching you! Don't be afraid to remind them to do this.

❑ Don't be afraid to cough. Coughing is good post-op; it reduces your risk of pulmonary complications.

❑ Do not stress out when you're having your surgical sutures removed. It really doesn't hurt! If you feel very anxious, do some deep breathing, breathing in through your nose and out through your mouth. Plan your pain medication to coincide with the timing of the removal, taking your medication about 45 minutes before removal. Take a whiff of lavender to relax you.

❑ Ask if your doctor will be willing to give you your prescriptions for post-op medications a day or two before surgery (or discharge, if you are being hospitalized) so you can have them in the house upon your arrival home from the hospital. Keep your medications nearby once you go home so they are easily accessible to you.

❑ Don't go home without discussing post-op bowel function with your doctor, especially if you tend to be constipated. Find out what you can use, and use it!

❑ If you are hospitalized, plan to take your last dose of pain medication about 45 minutes before you leave the hospital for home. It will help ease the discomfort during the ride home.

❑ Have a pillow in the car for the ride home from the hospital. It will help you position your knee more comfortably.

Once you are home:

❑ Follow all of your doctor's instructions!

❑ Don't be afraid to speak with your doctor about pain management. Icing helps a lot. Don't be a martyr. You don't need to suffer. Take your pain medications as prescribed for at least the first 2 weeks. It's important to stay on top of the pain. You may even want to set your alarm so you can keep on top of the pain during the night. This will actually help you recover more quickly, as your body can focus on healing, not on coping with pain. Keep your pain medications and water close by so you can easily reach them. Do not drive or operate any dangerous equipment or machinery while taking pain medications.

Narcotic pain medication prescriptions cannot be refilled or re-ordered over the phone. You will need to have someone go to your doctor's office to pick up a new prescription. Be sure to have enough pain medication in hand to cover your pain needs for any weekends or holidays when your doctor's office may be closed.

❑ Let your doctor know if you are having trouble sleeping. Adequate rest is important for you. You may be a good sleeper, but once you stop taking the narcotic pain medications, you might have trouble falling asleep.

❏ Use pillows to help yourself get comfortable at night. A pillow under your knees may also help you get more comfortable. Speak to your surgeon about pillows.

❏ Make a list of any questions you might want to ask your doctor at your first post-op visit, which usually takes place 7–10 days after surgery. If you had sutures, they will probably be removed at this visit.

Time your pain medication so you take it about 45 minutes prior to any outing.

Physical therapy is critical to your complete recovery! It is no picnic, but you must actively participate. Take your pain medication about 45 minutes prior to physical therapy. This will help maximize your therapy session. Don't expect an overnight recovery.

Call your doctor immediately if you have any of the following symptoms:

❏ Fever

❏ Sweats

❏ Redness around or drainage from your incision

❏ Shaking chills

FREQUENTLY ASKED QUESTIONS

1. **How do I get my medical bills paid?**

    Your Patient Bill of Rights states that you have the right to full infor-
    mation and counseling about the availability of known financial
    resources for your health care. Talk to your hospital's financial coun-
    selor to manage and pay your bills. The bill cannot be ignored.

2. **What if my doctor is not meeting my needs?**

    First, ask yourself if you are being a "good" patient. Are you arriving
    on time for appointments, paying your bills in a timely manner, fol-
    lowing the doctor's instructions? If you are a "good" patient and you
    just don't feel comfortable with the doctor, be assertive and have a
    conversation with the doctor about your concerns. If that fails to
    change your perception of how you are being treated, you may
    decide to change doctors. You have a voice. ... Use it!

3. **What should I bring with me when I'm being admitted to the
    hospital?**

    Be sure to bring your health insurance card(s) in addition to past
    and current health information and medical history. Bring your
    medication containers or a list of current medications you are on.
    Bring copies of your health care advance directives. Bring a bag of
    personal items that you will need, including slippers that are easy
    to slip on, and a pair of inexpensive flip-flops for taking showers. If
    you are having surgery, be sure to bring loose-fitting clothing to
    wear on your way home. Bring a certificate showing if you donated
    your own blood for your surgical procedure. Bring the names and
    phone numbers of family and friends. Bring paper and pencil with

you so you can write down all of your questions that need to be answered. Leave all valuables at home.

4. **Will hospice dignify my dying husband's remaining days?**

    Most families who have experienced hospice care of a loved one will share beautiful and heartwarming stories about their hospice experience and the "angels" who do the very holy work of caring for the terminally ill with compassion and love. Be assured your husband's hospice team will use whatever appropriate treatment and comfort measures they can as they dignify death and support your husband and your entire family in the process.

5. **My father is dying. What should I expect from the hospital nurses caring for him?**

    They will use whatever appropriate treatment and comfort measures they can as they dignify death and support your father and the entire family in the process.

6. **How do I prepare for a doctor visit?**

    Make a list of all the symptoms you have been having. Bring your health insurance ID card with you. Either bring a written list (including the doses) or the containers of all the medications that you are currently taking. This includes any herbs, supplements, vitamins, and other over-the-counter (OTC) drugs. Bring all of your past and current health information. This includes the written results of any lab or diagnostic tests you may have taken. Bring an advocate with you—family or friend. Research any pertinent medical issues on the internet so you have some knowledge of your medical status. Provide your doctor with your health care advance directive.

7. **When should I go to the emergency room?**

    You should call 911 for any of the following conditions: chest pain, heart attack or suspected heart attack, poisoning, severe shortness of breath, uncontrolled or severe bleeding, suspected overdose of medication, severe burns, high fever (especially in infants), loss of consciousness, head injury, seizures, diabetic complications such as insulin shock or diabetic ketoacidosis, gunshot or stab wounds, severe and persistent abdominal pain.

8. **My husband is not the same person he was before his stroke. When will he return to being himself?**

    Doctors will be unable to accurately predict the actual outcome of the brain injury resulting from the stroke your husband suffered. Even with the slightest of injuries, there can be subtle changes in the patient's personality, intellectual functioning, or mental state. Life with your husband as you have known it has changed, and getting it back to exactly where it was prior to the accident is unlikely.

9. **I'm having a colonoscopy. Will it hurt?**

    You will be given medications throughout the procedure. You will neither feel nor remember what takes place.

10. **How are my privacy and confidentiality guaranteed in the health care setting?**

    HIPAA, the Health Information Portability and Accountability Act of 1996, protects your personal information by holding *everyone* who works in the health care setting ethically and legally responsible for maintaining your confidentiality.

11. **Why do I need a patient advocate?**

    As a patient, you absorb a lot less information when you are anxious, vulnerable, in pain, afraid, or undressed. In addition, there are times when you may not be able to speak for yourself, such as when you are scared, anxious, in pain, unconscious, under sedation or anesthesia, or disabled, to name a few.

12. **What do I need to know when my doctor wants me to have a diagnostic test?**

Many questions need to be asked when your physician has suggested some diagnostic testing. These are the three most important ones: What is my main problem? What do I need to do? Why is it important for me to do this?

13. **I need copies of my medical records. How can I get access to them?**

According to the Patient Bill of Rights, the facility is required to provide you or your patient designee, upon request, access to all information contained in your medical records. You are also entitled to have copies of all of your medical records. Start with your bedside nurse. If necessary, call for the nursing supervisor or hospital administrator.

14. **I've moved to a new city. How do I find a doctor?**

Call your local hospital or ask people you meet for referrals.

15. **Why won't my doctor prescribe antibiotics when I have the flu?**

Antibiotics are used to treat bacterial infections. The flu is caused by a virus.

16. **I have heard about a new spinal surgery that does not involve cutting into the spine. What is this surgery called, and how is it performed?**

A new minimally invasive endoscopic procedure is now being done. An endoscopic tube is inserted through a tiny incision. Using a microscopic camera, the surgeon can repair the spine. Be sure to ask your orthopedic surgeon if he or she performs such surgery.

17. **My father is being discharged from the hospital after a one-month hospitalization. I know he will require care once he's home. How will I manage that?**

The hospital discharge planning nurse and social worker will be involved with this. They will make arrangements for a home health nurse to visit your father's home after discharge to do an initial evaluation, determine needs, and plan accordingly. If your father has home health or long-term care insurance, be sure to share that with all involved. You can also notify the insurance carriers on your own to start the ball rolling.

18. **My mother is dying and my family has yet to discuss her inevitable death with her. My brother says we should not have this conversation with her. I feel she deserves that conversation. Who is right?**

You are correct. If you ignore the inevitability of death and do not have this important conversation with your loved one, you leave that person alone to face this most difficult final journey without the requisite love and support so critical to a peaceful passing. There is nothing worse than facing the end of your life with everyone around you pretending that it is not happening.

19. **My husband's father and brother both died from prostate cancer before age seventy. Should we expect my husband to die from this disease as well?**

While prostate cancer does run in families, your husband's fate from the same illness is not inevitable. He should be sure to have a physical exam each year (or more often), which includes a Prostate Specific Antigen blood test (PSA). That simple blood test and physical exam can detect disease in its early stages and give him his best hope for a complete cure.

20. **The specialist my primary physician referred me to makes me feel really uncomfortable and stupid. What should I do?**

Most health care consumers prefer to use doctors who make them feel warm and fuzzy. This is fine, but there might be times when you have to forgo the warm heart for a smart brain. Do not be embarrassed to change doctors when the one you are currently using is not meeting all of your needs. It happens every day. Be assertive and proactive for yourself. You have a voice. ... Use it!

21. **Do I have the right to refuse prescribed treatment in the hospital?**

    Yes, you have the right to refuse treatment or care in the hospital. Be sure to tell the health care worker why you are refusing so he or she can understand. In turn, you need to understand the consequences of that refusal. The financial consequence is that your insurance company may refuse to pay for your hospitalization if you continually refuse care.

22. **I suffer from chronic back pain. A friend has recommended I see an acupuncturist. Is this something that I should pursue?**

    Although seeking out alternative or complementary medical treatment may be a good thing, it should be used as an adjunct along with standard conventional medical treatment. Discuss this alternative or complementary treatment with your personal doctor.

23. **My friend is dying. I am hesitant to visit her because I don't know what to say and I am afraid I will say the wrong thing and upset her.**

    Go visit your friend! She needs you now more than ever. Tell her you don't know what to say but you are there because you care and you'll be with her throughout her journey. These are very comforting words for a terminally ill patient to hear. Often, dying patients don't even want to talk. They just want to know that people care.

24. **My young adult daughter is in the hospital. She is on medication that makes her groggy. I want to be involved with her care but don't know what I should do.**

    If you accept this advocacy role, you should plan on being with your loved one as much as possible. Use your voice to ask about diagnosis, prognosis, medications, and diagnostic tests. Ask the questions that your loved one is unable to ask for herself, and be sure to share the answers with her when she is able to understand.

25. What do I need to know before signing a consent for surgery?

Before you sign the consent form for any invasive procedure, be sure your doctor has explained the procedure to you. Just like with any legal contract, you should read the fine print, the "Terms and Conditions of Service." Do not let anyone rush you through this process, putting you under pressure to sign something you haven't had time to digest or understand. Seek information if you don't understand what you're signing. As with all legal documents, changes can be legally made to the contract by using a single horizontal line to cross out what you do not agree with, by initialing the change, and by writing what you desire regarding that change on the bottom of the form.

NOTES

_____

_____

_____

_____

_____

_____

_____

_____

_____

_____

_____

_____

_____

_____

YOU HAVE A VOICE... USE IT!

NOTES

_____

_____

_____

_____

_____

_____

_____

_____

_____

_____

_____

_____

_____

YOU HAVE A VOICE... USE IT!

NOTES

_____

_____

_____

_____

_____

_____

_____

_____

_____

_____

_____

_____

_____

_____

YOU HAVE A VOICE... USE IT!

NOTES

_____

_____

_____

_____

_____

_____

_____

_____

_____

_____

_____

_____

_____

_____

YOU HAVE A VOICE... USE IT!

NOTES

_____

_____

_____

_____

_____

_____

_____

_____

_____

_____

_____

_____

_____

YOU HAVE A VOICE... USE IT!

NOTES

_____

_____

_____

_____

_____

_____

_____

_____

_____

_____

_____

_____

_____

_____

YOU HAVE A VOICE... USE IT!

MY MEDICATION CHART

DRUG	DOSE	SIDE EFFECTS	WHICH DR. PRESCRIBED IT?	WHY AM I TAKING IT?	WHAT DOES THE PILL LOOK LIKE?

MY MEDICATION CHART

DRUG	DOSE	SIDE EFFECTS	WHICH DR. PRESCRIBED IT?	WHY AM I TAKING IT?	WHAT DOES THE PILL LOOK LIKE?		

CPSIA information can be obtained
at www.ICGtesting.com
Printed in the USA
FFOW01n1123101117
43246457-42012FF